Change Works with CLEAR℠
Clearing Limits Energetically with Acupressure Release

Julie Roberts, Ph.D.
© August 21, 2006

Table of Contents

Acknowledgments — v

Preface — 1

CHAPTER 1: Overview of CLEAR — 3
What is CLEAR? — 3
What can CLEAR do for me? — 4
    Even though I can't have a relationship…. — 4
    Even though I don't deserve lots of money… — 5
    Even though I have to be the responsible one, and I don't deserve to take care of myself… — 7

CHAPTER 2: What is trauma, and how does CLEAR help? — 11
    Even though I get depressed when it's hot and humid… — 11
    What does CLEAR do? — 12
    How does CLEAR work? — 12
    How is this method different? — 14
    Using CLEAR — 14

CHAPTER 3: Understanding Trauma — 17
    Stress — 19
    Symptoms of trauma — 19
    Allergies — 20
    Blocking beliefs — 21

Feeling our emotions	22
Muscle testing	24

CHAPTER 4: Working with Children — 27
Sam: Letting go of acting out	27
Andrew: Releasing the negative impacts of a car accident	28
Benefits of CLEAR when working with children	29

CHAPTER 5: How Behavioral Change Works in the CLEAR Process — 31
Sarah: Changing patterns of abuse	31
William: Changing old habits	32
David: Re-traumatizing ourselves with our own behavior	33

HOW TO SECTION — 35

CHAPTER 6: Using Muscle Testing — 37
Muscle testing others	37
Self-testing	38
Creating statements to use in muscle testing	39

CHAPTER 7: The Steps in the CLEAR Process — 41
A note about the impact of working with people	41
Step 1: Identifying the issue	41
Step 2: Reversals	43
Step 3: Muscle testing	44
Flow chart	45
Outline for clearing	46
Step 4: Clearing blocking beliefs	47
Step 5: Clearing the points	48
Focus when clearing	49
The body	49
Origins	49
Healed version	50

Step 6: Blocking beliefs on the issue	51
Emotions and blocking beliefs	52

CHAPTER 8: Learning the Acupressure Points — 55
- Acupressure point table — 56
- Acupressure point illustrations — 58

CHAPTER 9: Sample session — 61

APPENDIX A: The Evolution of Acupressure Point Energy Therapy — 75

APPENDIX B: The Underlying Principles of Energy Work — 79
- We are all connected — 79
- There is enough to go around — 82
- We create our reality — 83
- Thankfulness and forgiveness — 84
- The importance of emotions — 85
- Understanding love and fear — 87
- Alignment is critical — 88
- The power of the past — 89
- Becoming conscious of our impact — 90
- Illuminating the energetic body — 91
- The fundamental paradoxes by which we evolve — 92
- We are all evolving — 92

APPENDIX C: Specific Blocking Beliefs — 93
- Being in love blocking beliefs — 93
- Belonging blocking beliefs — 94
- Connection blocking beliefs — 94
- Female blocking beliefs — 95
- Male blocking beliefs (females may have these also) — 96
- Money blocking beliefs — 96
- Over-responsibility — 97
- Religion related blocking beliefs — 98

Relationship blocking beliefs	98
Responsibility blocking beliefs	99
Self-Love blocking beliefs	99
Work and success blocking beliefs	99
APPENDIX D: Useful Exercises	**101**
The waterfall exercise	101
Being present in your body	101
Breathing through the heart	102
Loving self exercise	102
APPENDIX E: Issues Cleared	**103**
Work and career	103
Self-concept	103
Family issues	104
Relationships	104
Emotions	104
Sex	105
Sleep	105
Miscellaneous	105
Bibliography	**107**
About the Author	**109**

Acknowledgments

I would like to thank all of my friends, as well as the students and clients of the energy therapies, without whom this book would not have materialized. They helped me to clarify and simplify the process, and they encouraged me to continue writing. It is through my clients that the work has evolved; their sessions provided the valuable examples in the book.

Thank you Rod Napier, for your initial suggestions and your ongoing support for this work. You are my biggest fan.

Particularly, thanks to April Heaslip for your loving nudges, checking in, and for bringing yourself and Rose Watson to my house to help me convey more of my own voice. Rose, you brought new life to the examples. April, I'm sorry I didn't completely remove all of the "shoulds." And thank you Joyce Ferris, for your appreciation and suggestions, and Olivia Rud for your marketing advice.

Thank you Susan Watrous, for your excellent editing job. Your suggestions regarding organization and flow added elegance to the writing. And thank you for introducing me to Melody Chu, who did an excellent job in formatting and designing the book.

Thank you Les Daroff, for turning me on to this work. And to my friends David Baum and David Knudsen, thank you for your honesty, encouragement and support on my journey.

Jason Shulman, my Kabbalah teacher, drove home the importance of being present in one's body.

My parents supported all of the careers I've chosen and instilled values of acceptance, continuous learning, love of the earth, and personal growth—thank you Mom and Dad.

My animals—Rio, Radar, Scout and Kirby—provide unconditional love, and the land and spirit nourish me.

Preface

When I was eleven, my parents threw their yearly Christmas party. The Christmas tree, which reached the peak of the cathedral ceiling, shimmered with lights, decorations, and tinsel. Memory tells me that someone slipped me some spiced eggnog, and as a result, I was sitting quietly on our orange, imitation-leather couch eavesdropping on the adults. This kind of thoughtful surveillance wasn't my usual MO at eleven, but that night contemplative observation offered a valuable and lifelong lesson.

Several adults were involved in an animated discussion. I don't remember the content of the conversation, and I am not sure I understood it even then, but I do know that one of the adults was acting in a way that seemed very childish, even to me. He was red in the face, pushy, argumentative, and forceful, almost like he was having a tantrum. He wasn't listening, and didn't seem to care what others were saying. I was shocked. How could an adult be acting this way? My world tilted and all my beliefs about growing up shifted. Apparently, growing up did not guarantee that one acted "grown up." It was an understanding that frightened and motivated me. I knew as sure as I knew I was sitting on the couch that I would have to work to grow up. And I have been loyal to that cause and improving myself diligently ever since.

CHAPTER 1
Overview of CLEAR

What is CLEAR?

Clearing Limitations Energetically with Acupressure Release is one of the methods called "energy psychology." These methods are profound and powerful processes for creating personal change that are relatively new in the field of counseling and psychology. Whether people want to ease emotional pain, relieve anxiety, free themselves of depression or a lack of motivation, this therapeutic technique clears the negative programming that leads to these states. Negative states limit our potential. Releasing the origins of the condition helps us improve our lives in many ways, resulting in more contentment, less stress, improved physical and emotional health, and the ability to change ineffective patterns.

Energy psychology evolved from the observation that specific acupuncture points are related to particular emotions. Practitioners noted that stimulating a point releases chemicals in the brain, which relieves negative feelings. Thus, CLEAR evolved from a number of the acupressure methods and a few other energy therapies (see Appendix A). Later in the book, you'll find more details of how and why the process works, but for now, know that you can find relief from your symptoms quickly and completely using this technique.

CLEAR dramatically cuts treatment time and offers results that are superior to traditional talk therapy. Some clients only use the process a few times. I remember one young woman who came to me very depressed. We did one, two-hour session. I didn't hear from her for two weeks, which worried me, so I called her to check in. She said she was happy and had no more depression. And after only one session! In traditional therapy, this woman would no doubt have been put on antidepressants and seen a therapist frequently for a much longer period of time.

Change Works with CLEAR

Some of my clients, students and I use the process regularly when issues arise that negatively impact our ability to be who we want to be and accomplish our goals. Changes take place immediately. Clients feel better in one to six sessions as opposed to years in traditional therapy. The process clears the origin of ineffective states or behaviors, so the system is no longer wired to respond in predictable and unproductive ways.

Anyone can use CLEAR, either on themselves or with others. You do not have to be a trained professional to experience the benefits of this method. This book leads you through precise steps to feel results immediately.

What can CLEAR do for me?
CLEAR helps in a variety of situations, including when:
- You feel blocked in your ability to create the life you want;
- You feel negatively affected in the present by past issues;
- You are depressed, unhappy, lack motivation, or procrastinate;
- You are overly anxious, frustrated or angry;
- You are afraid to fly;
- You want to free up your potential, your creativity and your intelligence.

In this chapter, I provide three examples from my work with clients that illustrate the CLEAR process and the kinds of issues you can address. Later, I'll explain the CLEAR process in detail, referencing elements from these examples.

"Even though I can't have a relationship…."
One young man we'll call Simon came to see me because he wanted to change some foundational elements of his life. For example, he was thirty-something, yet had never had a girlfriend. This surprised me because he was quite good-looking and very fit. Speaking in short, clipped sentences, Simon said he had no friends to speak of either. He gave little detail and in order to draw him out, I asked focused questions about his life and relationships. Here were some of the things he said in the beginning of our session:

Overview of CLEAR

- I feel out of place.
- I don't know how to get "in."
- I don't fit in.
- My parents considered the people around me weird.
- I don't trust other people's judgment.
- Others won't measure up.
- I want to keep my distance.
- I'm different and out of place.
- They aren't interested in me.
- I don't get what they see in me.
- I'm not loveable.
- I may lose my identity if I connect with them.

Are you wondering how Simon could have a relationship if he believed these things? They are blocking beliefs that developed from his life experience. For example, imagine the impact of his parents saying that his friends were weird every time he brought someone home. Can you see how he might feel out of place, isolated and alone?

For the purpose of working with CLEAR, it doesn't matter how these beliefs came about. Even though I learned more about Simon's history as we worked together what I listened for as he spoke were the beliefs (e.g., "I don't fit in") and issues (e.g., "I feel out of place") that, when cleared, will free him to have the relationships he wants.

Simon and I worked together for one, two-hour session in which he released his blocking beliefs. We cleared how he felt out of place, his judgments, and his fears about being connected to others. A few weeks after this session, I called to check in with him. Speaking with obvious pride and pleasure, he reported that he had a new girlfriend and he was hanging out with a group of people from work. I was thrilled that the changes that he sought were occurring!

Even though I don't deserve lots of money...

Over the years of using the energy therapies I have witnessed people create miraculous changes. Diane was one of those. When we met, she reported that she was struggling with financial issues. Her car was unreliable, and she felt constantly stressed about having enough money. We dedicated a whole session to the issue of money. She had some common blocking beliefs about the topic, such as:

- I can't have lots of money and be a spiritual person.
- Money is evil.
- It's a sin to have money.
- Money is the root of all evil.
- It's greedy to want things I don't have.
- It is selfish to want it.
- I don't deserve lots of money.
- In order to have money I have to work really hard.
- It's not possible to have lots of money.
- I'm not smart enough to make lots of money.
- People won't like me if I have lots of money.

On a Thursday, we cleared her blocking beliefs and issues related to deprivation and deserving abundance. That Friday Diane went to her mother's for a visit and her mother gave her a bag full of money, which Diane used to buy a new car. When she went to work the following Monday, her supervisor said Diane was getting a raise. Is this a miracle? Coincidence? My hypothesis is that the effect of changing one's belief and energetic system results in changes in the physical world. When we feel worthy of that which we desire, and there are no related blocking beliefs, it is more likely that our dreams will manifest. If we believe at any level, for any reason that we don't deserve or want something, then chances are that thing will not end up in our lives. Or it will end up in our lives in a way that is not helpful, or is challenging instead of simply beneficial. Take, for example, a 25-year-old acquaintance of mine who has difficulty with money. She never has enough, and always feels resentful that she doesn't have enough because she was given a trust fund by a wealthy relative, which she won't be able to access until she turns 50. Because she knows she will eventually have plenty of money, she waits for the day she turns 50. She doesn't want to work or pursue a career because she knows at 50, she will no longer have to work. Meanwhile, 25 years of her life are spent in this limbo-land where she waits for life to begin.

Overview of CLEAR

An issue like money is often complex. I have seen clients work on money in different ways in many sessions because it is such a core issue with so much related to it in terms of history, survival, and sustenance.

Change using the CLEAR method is not always as immediate as it was for Diane and Simon, however, when you have blocks like theirs, you can release them, usually in one to six sessions of working with CLEAR. When a client returns for a second session, I ask him or her to review the issues cleared in the previous visit. As they do, they usually report that they are doing things differently. Many people say they feel "lighter" or more peaceful after a session, and note that their lives are moving in a positive direction, often without much effort.

Periodically, a client doesn't think that CLEAR works for him because he doesn't feel any differently after a session. Yet when I ask him how he feels and is dealing with the issue we cleared, he feels and is doing things differently around an issue. For example, one man who is a consultant, became anxious when he saw that he didn't have work scheduled in the months ahead. In reality, he was always fine over time, but when he didn't have work, he got stressed and worried. We cleared issues around being secure, having enough, and being competent, and he stopped having the anxiety. He didn't think the energy therapies had worked for him, but when I asked why he was feeling differently around his work schedule, he said he just figured he had changed. I mentioned that we had cleared this and perhaps it was related to the clearing. He agreed that I was probably right.

Even though I have to be the responsible one and I don't deserve to take care of myself...

When Jane, 55, came to see me she suffered from extreme anxiety. Her drawn, pale face was pinched in an almost-perpetual worried frown. She felt overly responsible and was exhausted, often feeling like she couldn't cope. She was doing too much at her job. She said she wanted to admit herself to an old folks home so that she could just sit and do nothing. Jane was so exhausted and burned out that she wanted no responsibility and no interactions with anyone.

We explored her sense of responsibility, clearing many blocking beliefs related to that issue. We cleared trauma resulting from her incomplete connections with her parents, and the loss of her grandparents. The "Over-responsibility" and "Connection" blocking beliefs in Appendix C began with Jane.

She also had a very difficult time throwing anything out, so her house was cluttered and overflowing. This was very frustrating for her because she understood feng shui and the potential negative impact of her clutter. She was attached to many things. Moreover, she believed that she needed to keep things given to her by people she loved because if she got rid of the thing, she lessened her emotional connection to that person. It was as though she would be disloyal to them, even if they were dead, if she got rid of the gift. All of the following beliefs and their related traumas, we cleared in about six sessions, spread over about six months:

- I have to take care of everyone.
- I'm overwhelmed.
- I have to be the responsible one.
- I can't do it all.
- It's not safe to get help from others.
- If I let go of my sad feelings (re: my parents' death), I won't be able to connect to them.
- I'll lose my connection to them if I lose objects related to them.
- I have to be on alert all the time to protect myself.
- I can never please my father.
- I'm afraid to connect.
- I'll be turned away.
- It's not right to connect with myself.
- I've got to do their thing, not my thing.

After each session Jane and I witnessed some progress, and by the end of six months (she saw me about once a month) she was relaxed, not taking on too much work, enjoying life, feeling like she could cope, and taking boxes of "stuff" to the Salvation Army. Jane was really becoming the person she wanted to be.

• • •

Overview of CLEAR

Whether you feel stuck in your life or just know there is more that you can accomplish, this book will assist you. CLEAR helps you move toward your goals by removing triggers that keep you stuck in old patterns. It helps relieve general and specific anxiety as well as specific issues such as phobias, performance anxiety, and test anxiety. It helps remove stress that leads to illness. It also assists you in clearing the blocks that lead to procrastination, lack of motivation, and fears related to success and failure. CLEAR alleviates depression and moodiness, and helps you understand the issues underlying these emotions.

CLEAR is for professionals and lay people. Anyone who wants to create change and is serious about changing can use this process. I wrote *Change Works* for people who want to create change for themselves or facilitate the possibility of change with others. You can do CLEAR by yourself or with the help of a partner.

My goal in writing this book is to make CLEAR available to everyone. It is an amazing process, and I hope it helps many people as it has helped me, my clients, and friends.

CHAPTER 2
What is Trauma and how does CLEAR Help?

Do you react emotionally to the weather, or a sound, or even a special smell? Will someone's particular word or expression send you into a seemingly uncontrollable negative spiral? Often a traumatic event in the distant past triggers these cascades of automatic reactions. Removing the trauma associated with the initial experience also removes the trigger and frees you from the reactions. Let's look at Sarah's case as an example of how this works.

Even though I get depressed when it's hot and humid…

As summer approached, Sarah was hardly able to function normally because of her anxiety. Twenty years prior, on a hot, humid evening, she had been attacked in her home. Since that trauma, she experienced deep depression every summer when the weather became muggy. She felt insecure and trapped in her life, and she didn't trust anyone. Though beautiful, kind and intelligent, she felt little confidence in herself.

Over a series of six sessions, we worked on and cleared the event when she was attacked, as well as related traumas from her past—that is, any event that reminded her of the unsafe feelings she had as a result of the attack, and any beliefs and trauma that resulted from the break-in:
- I have to stay inside.
- I am not safe.
- I'm trapped.
- I'll be hurt.
- People aren't safe.
- I shouldn't be around people.

The last time I saw her (her sixth session), she said, "This is the first time in 20 years that I have not gone into a deep depression when the hot, humid weather hit." Sarah cleared this trauma and surrounding issues at an energetic level using CLEAR, which freed her from the link her body had with the weather.

What does CLEAR do?

CLEAR helps to change your beliefs. By accelerating the process of change, CLEAR makes traditional talk therapy more effective and realistic. Moreover, CLEAR frees you from ineffective patterns and helps integrate new effective behaviors. Using the CLEAR process helps actualize your potential, removes blocks, and aids you in accessing your spiritual connection.

One of the most powerful ways that CLEAR works to bring you more fully into the present moment is by removing past and future anxieties. By alleviating trauma and negative beliefs, you move forward in your life. For example, in the case study in chapter 1, Jane experienced situations that led her to believe that she was the only person who could be responsible and that "it was all up to her." Once she cleared the trauma behind this and its associated beliefs, she could relax and let others do some of the work. In Sarah's case, we cleared a twenty-year problem of seasonally associated depression in six sessions. This is a problem she was not able to remedy with talk therapy.

Working at the traditional levels in therapy (intellectual, emotional, physical, behavioral) is slow and time consuming. CLEAR works at the energetic level, which is faster and usually heals all of the other levels at the same time. Clearing trauma and beliefs frees up people to respond differently. Often after a single session, clients see new ways of responding spontaneously, and wonder why they never thought of responding that way before.

How does CLEAR work?

Clearing Limits Energetically with Acupressure Release uses acupressure points to free issues that negatively impact your life. The client touches an acupressure point while thinking of the problem. During reprocessing you remain present in your body and experience your thoughts, emotions, and bodily sensations while focusing on the issue being cleared. Muscle testing is then used to determine in which point (or points) the trauma resides, and then if the issue is cleared.

The process I describe in this book leads you through healing that frees you of old patterns, allowing you to be present to your current thoughts and feelings, and thus more creative in your responses.

Acupressure points, when stimulated by touching, rubbing or tapping, transmit signals directly to the specific areas of the brain that are associated with those emotions. Research has found that the stimulation of the point inhibits the "alarm response" by sending appropriate signals directly to the amygdala (Feinstein, Eden & Graig, 2005). Ronald Ruden, M.D., Ph.D., states that stimulation of acupressure points increases serotonin in the cortex and the amygdala, thus removing fear and shifting negative responses to positive ones (Ruden, 2005). Studies using brain scans also indicate a significant decrease in intensity and frequency of Generalized Anxiety Disorder after acupressure treatment (Andrade, & Feinstein 2003).

Feinstein, in *The Promise of Energy Psychology*, states that the energy therapies "…help a person overcome that problem or reach that goal by changing the chemistry in the amygdala and other areas of the brain". Observing my clients, I see that there is indeed a positive change resulting in a rewiring of the brain that removes the automatic response to a stimulus.

An important note here: It is not necessary to *re-live* the trauma to work with it. But in this experience of reprocessing and remaining in the body physically and emotionally, the person finishes processing the trauma and can free it from the body. The bodily reactions necessary for reprocessing arise naturally during the process.

Typically, clients notice changes or feel progress after each session, and the more issues they clear, the more progress they make in terms of where they want to go and how they want to be in the world. Thus, clients move toward their goals, a sense of peace, and the easing of issues that were formerly so present in their lives.

Change Works with CLEAR

How is this method different?

The method described in this book is different from other energy therapies in a number of ways. First, there is no "tapping" required as in some of the other acupressure methods. Instead, clients touch, gently tap, or rub the point. There is no need to check on Subjective Units of Disturbance ("SUDs") where the client rates the emotion she is feeling on a scale of one to ten. Instead, I use muscle testing to see if the issue is clear. When an issue hasn't been released, I repeat the muscle testing to isolate the related blocking beliefs or trauma, which we then clear.

Many energy therapies use a given sequence of points that the client repeats for every issue. Instead, I teach a process that is guided by client's needs, and which tracks the process. I provide instructions for customizing the steps to the client's particular issues. For this reason, this process is also more efficient than many other methods.

This methodology assumes that blocking beliefs play a large part in the healing process, and that clearing them is critical to releasing past issues that negatively impact our lives. Clients clear anywhere from five to fifty or more blocking beliefs related to one issue. This method is thorough. Sometimes it can take considerable focus to follow an issue through to the final clearing, but with the help of muscle testing and good notes, you can easily track the issue and permanently and completely clear it.

Using CLEAR

How often do I use CLEAR? With some clients—for example, Simon—one session of CLEAR is enough. Some use it initially to clear an issue they know is blocking them in their lives, and then continue to use it to deal with concerns as they arise, as in the case of Sarah. I, and those who study with me, use it whenever blocks become evident. For example, as I began this book, I realized that an incident with a previous editor on a different book was blocking me from moving forward. After I cleared the issue, I found myself writing easily and moving forward with the book. Often, as we live our lives, we find that past experience is inhibiting our momentum. This is a good time to use this process to check for and clear issues that may be blocking us.

If you are working with the CLEAR process by yourself, you split your attention between what you feel and think, and at the same time you listen for what needs clearing.

What is Trauma and how does CLEAR Help?

This becomes easier as you get more experience, but initially you may find it easier to work with a partner. Many of my clients who know how to use CLEAR on themselves still come to see me because then they can be fully present to feelings and what is going on in the body without having to pay attention to the issues and hear what needs to be cleared at the same time.

If you want to use CLEAR on others as a practitioner, I recommend that you work on yourself in order to work more effectively with others. The more you clear in yourself, the more you will be a clear and focused lens for others. Remember, when you work with others, you have a responsibility to be as present as possible with their issues, and understand when you are being activated by something on which the other person is working. If something they are working on triggers you, be sure to come back to that and work on it later on yourself.

Past trauma can cause difficult patterns and behaviors for us currently, but CLEAR helps free us of the beliefs and triggers to that behavior. The process of clearing may be emotional—or not. It is important to avoid expectations of how the clearing will look. It will be what it is, and the muscle testing will let you know if an issue effectively cleared or not.

CHAPTER 3
Understanding Trauma

As we have already seen, the experience of old trauma may prevent you from being fully present. Sarah, for example, couldn't be fully in the moment during the summer because the weather stimulated her past trauma of being attacked. Once the trauma was cleared, she could live without the depression that kept her from being present in her life.

This chapter elucidates trauma, and how we become traumatized. We'll explore common symptoms of trauma, allergies and their relation to trauma, and the impact of blocking beliefs, as well as learn about muscle testing and how it works.

Trauma may result from a physical experience such as a car accident, or from an emotional incident such as being attacked in your home as in the case of Sarah. It may be the result of living with irresponsible parents and feeling the need to take care of them, as with Jane. It may occur because of repetitive negative events such as being yelled at by an unhappy and angry parent. Or it may be the result of something hurtful someone once said such as declaring that you are ugly, stupid or ridiculous.

Peter Levine, the author of many books on the subject of trauma, observed animals in the natural world. If an animal, such as a deer, is attacked by a cougar, and can't fight or flee, it responds by going into the "immobility response." This response shuts down the system so the animal won't feel much pain when it is eaten. If the cougar is scared off for some reason, and the deer is not eaten, it will stay on the ground and twitch for a while before it gets up, shakes and runs off. According to Levine, the deer is processing the trauma and thus, the trauma doesn't get stuck in the deer's body.

Often humans don't fully process trauma, so it gets stuck in our bodies. People stop the body's natural processing of the trauma because of their *thoughts* about the *feelings* they have in traumatic situations. Traumatic situations don't feel good, so we try to escape from those feelings. We think, "I don't want to feel this way" that is, vulnerable or scared or hurt or unhappy, and we do whatever we can to avoid it. We certainly don't allow ourselves to lie there and twitch and role our eyes as an animal might after experiencing the immobility response. Yet escaping from the pain stops us from fully processing the trauma in the body, so it gets stuck in system.

Like other animals, people respond to any trauma with a hard-wired "fight-or-flight" response, and if we can't fight or flee, we too, go into the "immobility response." Fight, flight and immobility responses bypass the cognitive mind and we react to the potential danger before we even have time to think. All of these survival mechanisms protect us. It is obvious how the fight or flight keeps us safe: we are primed to run or fight the danger. The immobility response protects us, just as it does an animal, because it dulls our senses so that we don't feel much during the ordeal. If, for example, a parent hurts or abuses us, our senses are numbed and we don't feel the pain so intensely.

When the trauma gets stuck in the body, and we later witness a situation that reminds us of this past trauma, we react as though we are actually experiencing the trauma again, with the stressful response of flight-or-fight, or with the immobility response. Once we are "triggered" by a new event that resembles an old trauma, we have very little control over our behavior, thus we also have less access to our full potential for action, because we react from the old, reptilian, survival part of the brain. This situation could simply be a stressful condition that makes the body feel there is danger, and suddenly, we are reacting as though we are under attack. Unreleased trauma can control our behavior in ways that in the past kept us safe, but now limit us in our lives.

Our reactive behavior is usually a predictable response to the stuck trauma, such as withdrawing, being passive, attacking aggressively, spacing out, or disassociating. In other words, we do the same thing we always do when that trauma is triggered—whether the situation warrants this behavior or not. This response has, in the past, kept us safe. But it is a response that causes much stress, and is often not effective in the present because we are reacting from the old trauma and not to the current situation. As a result, we can be overly aggressive in a situation with a co-worker, thus alienating ourselves from others. Or we can space out whenever a big man like the boss comes into the room. Or we may just stay quiet. We don't risk putting ourselves out in a situation that seems threatening.

Each time we revisit the trauma, even just by thinking about it, we make the traumatic memory stronger (Johnson, 2004). This goes for "small" traumas as well as bigger ones. A "small" trauma may result from the comment your husband made about your lazy attempt to clean the floor yesterday, or it may be the near accident you had on the way home. But whatever the trauma, the more you think about it or talk about it without fully processing it in the body, the stronger you make the memory—and the more likely that you feel stress and anxiety as a result of it. It is for this reason that traditional talk therapy may not help trauma and care even make it worse.

Stress

Trauma causes stress. Every time we react with the fight-or-flight response or the immobility response, stress is the result. Part of us may think that trauma keeps us safe because it makes us vigilant to danger or it reminds us of what to watch out for, but stress is detrimental to the system and a precursor to heart attack. Stress produces adrenalin that increases heart rate and blood pressure, it causes the muscles to tighten, speeds up the breathing, and results in the release of cortisol. Chronically high levels of cortisol reduce immune function, increase bone loss, reduce muscle mass, increase fat accumulation, impair memory and learning, and destroy brain cells (Childre & Martin, 1999). The sense that trauma keeps us safe is actually an illusion. In fact, it prevents us from seeing reality clearly, and eventually causes disease. Clearly we benefit from clearing the traumas that cause our stress!

Symptoms of trauma

How do we know if trauma is stuck in our bodies? Peter Levine provides a wonderful list of the symptoms of trauma in his study guide to his "Healing Trauma" tapes. Symptoms of trauma that may follow shortly after the event include exaggerated startle response, nightmares, hyperactivity, mood swings, difficulty sleeping, and fear of losing sanity.

Later symptoms may include panic attacks, hypervigilance, anxiety, spacing out, avoidance, indulging in dangerous activities, mood swings, inability to bond with others, and a fear of dying. If the trauma is not cleared, symptoms later in life may include phobias, depression, inability to accomplish goals, and many physical disorders (such as stomach problems, chronic fatigue, asthma, allergies, immune system problems, thyroid, endocrine problems, and other vague or mysterious symptoms). CLEAR can remove these symptoms from the body. I have seen many people heal physical symptoms as a result of using the energy therapy.

One of my students worked with her seven-year-old son to see if she could help relieve his dizziness and blurry vision—one of those vague, mysterious, physical symptoms. He put his attention on the dizziness and blurry vision while pressing the appropriate acupressure points. It turns out he didn't want to say "no" to his teacher when he was presented with optional work. He didn't want to say no because he felt sorry for all the trees that were being wasted when she threw away the extra, unused pages. He thought it would be better if he did the work to save the paper. He and his mother cleared the points involved and discussed other ways he could recycle. Since then, the boy has had no dizziness or blurred vision.

Allergies

It is my theory, and others who work with energy psychology concur, that allergies are caused by the trauma we experience throughout our lives. When we clear trauma with the energy therapies, often people's allergies spontaneously disappear. It is also possible to work specifically on clearing allergies with positive results.

When we experience trauma, we most often have a visceral reaction of attempting to get away from or push away the situation and the things in the situation. We feel scared, repulsed, angry, and we want the stimulus to stop. This reaction actually causes the trauma to be registered in our system. Since our body is very literal, it determines that the situation and the things in it are not good for us and we need to get away from them.

We literally feel we need to create distance from the perceived threats in the situation in order to feel safe. Had I been beaten as a young child, for example, it is highly likely that I would be allergic to things that were around me when that occurred. If there was a lot of mold and dust in the house, then I may have allergies to them. If there were a dog or cat around, then I may have allergies to pets. Perhaps our bodies set up a warning signal: if I am around these things, then I will have a reaction telling me to get away. Or perhaps it is just a reaction where our bodies say, this is too much, I cannot handle any more of this thing, get me away, and the allergic reaction is a warning signal.

One of my clients I'll call Jessi was afraid she would have to get rid of her miniature poodle. She was having such a bad reaction to her dog, which she dearly loved, that she had to stay physically distant from her as much as possible; Jessi feared she'd even have to give the poodle away. When we initially discussed the issue, Jessi had no idea what traumas were related to her allergy, but during the session she made connections to particular traumas just by touching the points associated with her allergy. One of the related traumas that we cleared resulted from a past situation when she owned a difficult dog that she was unable to deal with, and so she had to get rid of it. She had guilt around abandoning the dog and felt that because she didn't keep it, she didn't deserve to have another dog. After this session (which we followed up with other sessions for other allergies), Jessi had no problem being around her dog, and actually was letting her dog sleep in the bed under the covers with her with no adverse reactions.

Blocking beliefs

As a result of stuck trauma, we develop what I call "blocking beliefs." A belief is a construct around which we live our lives, such as "I believe in God." A belief that results from trauma may be something like "I am not safe," or "Love hurts." If we believe, for example, that we aren't safe, then we live from that perspective, and consequently, we may avoid people or situations we believe are difficult or challenging.

Blocking beliefs protect us after a trauma. They are wired into us with the trauma to keep us safe. If I am hurt by someone, then I may have beliefs that I can't trust people, I'm not safe, and others will hurt me. Hypervigilance and anxiety can result from these beliefs.

Blocking beliefs are the beliefs within you, registered at an energetic level that prevent you from being who you desire to be fully. These beliefs exist because of what we are told as we go through life. And they arise as a result of the traumas we experience. Often a number of blocking beliefs exist around one specific issue. Detailed lists of common blocking beliefs are provided in Appendix C. Brief examples include "I'm not smart enough to succeed," or "I'll be hurt if I express my truth."

Blocking beliefs also protect us, as in the case of a belief like: "I have to be alert or I will be hurt," or "I will be hurt if I speak my mind." In an attempt to keep us safe, blocking beliefs are wired in with the trauma. The problem is that they also prevent us from responding in the moment with our full emotional and cerebral intelligence.

It is critical to the healing process to clear blocking beliefs. If a trauma is cleared without fully clearing the blocking beliefs associated with it, the trauma will not be completely cleared. Blocking beliefs are integrally linked to trauma and are, therefore, critical to understand and clear during the process. If I believe that the memory of a trauma keeps me safe, I will not effectively clear the trauma associated with that belief unless that belief is also cleared. For example, in the case of a woman who has been raped, often the woman believes that her hypervigilance keeps her safe. She thinks that if she clears the trauma, she won't be vigilant, and then danger may sneak in. Thus, the belief that the trauma keeps her safe needs to be cleared before the trauma is cleared.

As parents and caregivers, we can't completely protect our children from hearing and integrating negative messages, which result in blocking beliefs. We can't insulate them from potential traumas. And if, by some miracle, we do, be sure that society will find a way to influence their beliefs. Just think of the many messages children are bombarded with daily, such as, "I have to be bone-thin to be beautiful," or "Boys don't cry," or "Girls are emotional and weaker than boys."

The good news is that these beliefs can be cleared. To do this, two of the acupressure points (the "sore" points) are lightly massaged while repeating the belief. Beliefs are often linked with trauma, so it is important to clear the trauma also, but it can be cleared! The process for clearing blocking beliefs is described in the "How To" section of the book.

Feeling our emotions

"Without all of our emotions, we are not fully conscious."

Jason Shulman

It is important to remember that CLEAR does not rid us of our emotions. The CLEAR process clears trauma and eases pain from the past that may be impacting the current issue. Our emotions inform us. They are natural and necessary for our health. If we deny them, we are not fully present or conscious, and issues will again get stuck in the system because they are not fully processed. In this situation, illness may result.

If we feel sadness and loss due to a divorce or loss of a loved one, CLEAR may be helpful in clearing related past trauma and blocking beliefs that intensify our pain, or it may lessen our fear related to being alone and what will happen to us. But it is not a way to avoid feeling the pain of loss. Our emotions provide information and potential healing. They provide the opportunity for us to know ourselves. The learning that arises from a difficult situation where we feel our emotions may simply be that we recognize old trauma and blocking beliefs that we need to clear. Or it may be that the person with whom we are conversing expresses confusing messages that raise our anxiety. But ultimately, we won't understand why the emotions exist unless we let ourselves feel them.

The more we resist our emotions, the more likely that we create trauma in our efforts to get away from the feeling. It is not the emotion that causes trauma, but our reaction to it. If we are neutral regarding the feelings, then trauma is not stored in the system. Trauma is stored because of the desire to resist feeling what goes along with that trauma (fear, vulnerability, sadness, loss, confusion, and so on). If I am sad about the death of a friend, but I block the feelings, then I am in denial. This leads to blockage, which could lead to depression and eventually physical illness. This is the way that new experiences can become stuck in the system, which sends us once again into fight-or-flight or immobility in an attempt to keep us safe.

I have heard it said that when we are in denial we have two potential responses. We either respond with some form of spiritual disassociation, or we respond with violence. Either one of these is a form of acting out. Spiritual practice to disassociate from the pain is internal acting out, while violence is an external form of acting out.

Spiritual practice can be an attempt to escape from pain and the effects of trauma. Meditation produces calm and peacefulness. "I don't want to feel my pain, so I go to a place of serenity that I learned from spiritual exercises." This may exemplify some people's motivation for the practice. In many ways, of course, these are wonderful practices, but not as an attempt to *remove* oneself from pain. As my Kabbalah teacher, Jason Shulman said, rather than praying to God or spirit to remove my pain, I should be asking for help to feel my pain fully, for only then can I move through the emotions and prevent them from getting stuck in my system.

Denial of pain can also lead to violence when the feeling becomes so strong in the system that I respond to that feeling and act out on it. It is my belief that if our society developed more healthy beliefs about emotions (it is natural to cry; anger informs me; pain is natural; vulnerability is a path to understanding; it is good to feel my emotions), and if we encouraged responsibility/owning our feelings and full processing of emotions, it is probable that we would have less violence and brutality on this planet.

Accepting feelings seems like a contradiction; it is not easy to imagine having neutral feelings about and feeling accepting of emotions that are difficult to experience. But feeling the emotion without pushing it away allows the emotion to pass through us without creating more trauma. Imagine the body feeling relaxed while allowing/accepting the full depth of the emotion.

If I can feel the emotion and allow the resulting sensations in my body, I begin to understand how I feel and why I feel that way. In this process, I can express my feelings to others without acting out. The more transparent I am about why I feel the way I feel, the less conflict I will experience in my life. Thus, I can heal myself naturally and prevent further trauma in the future.

• • •

Muscle testing

Muscle testing (also referred to as Applied Kinesiology) is based upon the theory that our body subtly reacts to positive and negative stimulus. When the stimulus is positive, muscles remain strong, and when stimulus is negative, muscles have a weak reaction. There are "squeezometers" that measure the level of strength in a client's body by measuring the strength of her hand squeezing a machine. The more common way of using muscle testing is to have the person hold out her arm in front of her and parallel to the floor. You then push down on the arm while she resists (see "Muscle testing" in the "How To" section).

Some chiropractors use muscle testing to find the source of a weakness in the body. They touch a very particular point on the body that correlates with a particular part of the spine, while testing the arm. If the arm is weak (the muscle cannot hold firm) when the chiropractor pushes down on it, then the correlating spot on the spine needs adjustment. Some medical professionals use muscle testing to diagnose physical or dental problems. Some utilize the process to determine a patient's sensitivity to drugs or supplements. Other practitioners use it to test for allergies.

Muscle testing works just as well on emotional issues as it does on physical problems. Often the physical body responds more clearly and honestly through muscle testing than the logical or analytic mind does. The muscle testing process also provides answers from the body that are sometimes unavailable to the conscious mind.

In the CLEAR process, you will use muscle testing to test for trauma and blocking beliefs with a client. You will also use it to see which acupressure points to work on, and then to find out if the trauma is effectively cleared from the system.

As we have seen, muscle testing is useful in a variety of ways, both for gathering information about stored trauma in the body and for measuring the effectiveness of treatment.

CHAPTER 4
Working with Children

Children are very good subjects for CLEAR. Typically, they are less judgmental about the process, and have fewer blocking beliefs and traumas impacting their clearing. Trauma becomes more complex as we age both because we re-traumatize ourselves just by thinking about past traumas, and because new traumas occur that relate to old traumas, creating a complex web. Thus, sessions with children are usually shorter and less complicated than sessions with adults.

Sam: Letting go of acting out

Eight-year-old Sam was bright and handsome—a sort of very young Tom Cruise. Though he was small for his age, he held himself a bit aloof, like a tough, street-smart kid. Sam acted out in order to get attention. He believed that he was not smart and could not do well in school. He got into trouble because he fought with other boys in his class.

In a one-hour session we cleared these beliefs and the traumas surrounding them. Sam was an easy client. We started by clearing the beliefs that he was not smart:
- I am not smart.
- I'm not as smart as others.
- I can't keep up.
- Others do better than me.
- I can't read well.

There were also acupressure points to clear regarding this issue. The points were related to his anger at not being able to keep up; his shame and embarrassment at not being able to read like the other children; his fear of being left behind, and his need to feel strong.

After we worked with these initial beliefs and issues, we moved on to why Sam was fighting with other boys. We started with the acupressure points. He would hold the points while thinking about the incident. Periodically, he would share an insight he had, often about his parents and how he was mad at them for not letting him do what his friends were allowed to do, for example, watch violent movies or play violent computer games. I could see that Sam's anger at his parents motivated his fighting. Because he didn't deal directly with them about it—because he didn't know how—he acted out in school. We talked about ways that he could express his anger to his parents in a healthy way. If Sam could understand and express his anger, we could probably prevent future acting out in school. He agreed that he would try this, and at the end of the session, we discussed the issues with Sam's mother. They agreed to have regular times when they talked about what was bothering him.

The next time I saw Sam, this time to clear some trauma about an operation and medical tests he needed to have, his mother said his schoolwork had improved significantly and that he was getting along much better with his teacher and other students. There had been no incidents of fighting.

Andrew: Releasing the negative impacts of a car accident

When Andrew was nine, a car crashed into his mother's car on the passenger side where Andrew was sitting. He witnessed the woman in the other car smashing into the windshield and cutting her face. After the accident, driving with his mother caused stress for both of them; his fear and hypervigilance re-traumatized both himself and his mother. He inhaled sharply whenever a car came near them, and yelled at his mom to be careful and watch out for various things as she drove.

I spent about ten minutes with Andrew clearing the trauma. I asked him how he felt about driving. He said:
- Cars aren't safe.
- I'm not safe in a car.
- I have to watch everything to keep us safe.
- Driving is dangerous.

We cleared these beliefs by saying them as he rubbed his "sore spots." I then asked him to replay the accident in detail while he was touching the appropriate acupressure points. We only did two points and the muscle testing indicated that the incident was clear. I asked Andrew how he felt, and he said he felt good, relaxed. I remember wondering if that was it—if he could really be clear after only ten minutes. A week after the session, I talked with the Andrew's mother who reported he was now relaxed and back to his old self while driving in the car with her!

Benefits of CLEAR when working with children

A child doesn't have to share with you what is happening as he clears an issue, although it can be helpful if he does because you may hear blocking beliefs that need to be cleared. There are times when a child doesn't want to talk about what happened because it is too embarrassing or painful. The good news is that he doesn't have to share for CLEAR to work. If this is the case, you may want to create a list of beliefs that you think he might have as a result of the trauma, such as:

- I'm not safe.
- People aren't safe.
- I don't know what to do.
- I want to run away.

As you work through the session, clear those beliefs with him. Then you can muscle test for points to clear as explained in the "How to" section of the book.

One woman who trained with me used CLEAR with her seventeen-year-old son to relieve his test anxiety. As she worked with him, she realized that the process of listening, writing down what he said, and then repeating it back was extremely helpful in developing their relationship. The process helped her to be present with him in a non-judgmental way and allowed him to feel fully heard and understood. Incidentally, his test-taking abilities also improved.

In my experience, children usually like doing CLEAR. They seem comfortable and easy with the process, and will often ask to come back to see me because they can see the effects it has and they enjoy doing it.

CHAPTER 5
How Behavioral Change Works in the CLEAR Process

Often, if we want to create big changes in our lives, we must also change our behavior to avoid repeating and recreating old trauma. If, for example, our behaviors exhibit or set up an old, unhealthy pattern of behavior, we re-traumatize ourselves by behaving toward others in a way that is reminiscent of our old traumas. Thus, I often suggest behavioral change when I work with clients. Sarah's situation provides a vivid example of the way past problems can be displayed in behavior and re-traumatize a person.

Sarah: Changing patterns of abuse

As Sarah cleared much of her trauma and depression, she felt stronger and happier than she had in a 20 years, but she remained upset with her boyfriend. His episodic meanness came out in verbal abuse toward Sarah. She responded by being silent initially and then later lashing out. On a scale of ten, Sarah rated their relationship as a two in terms of her hope that it would survive. For the relationship to change, it seemed clear that Sarah must change her behavior toward this man.

Gradually, Sarah realized that her boyfriend's behavior was not acceptable. I suggested that she tell him she was upset in a calm and specific way, clearly describing the behavior she didn't like and explaining what she did want from him. Second, I suggested she examine her reactions to him because they kept her stuck in the pattern of abuse. By behaving the way others behaved toward her, she re-traumatized herself. Sarah agreed to try this change of behavior. She told her boyfriend that she did not want to be treated that way and would have to end it if things didn't change. He responded well, significantly changing his behavior. In a later visit with me, she said she gave the relationship an eight in terms of her hope for its survival.

In this case, the client had cleared the trauma of abuse, but her behavior kept her stuck in abusive situations and re-traumatized herself until she shifted her own behavior. When she began respecting herself and creating guidelines for what was acceptable and then communicated these guidelines to her boyfriend, things shifted. This was not a simple task, as she had to work against her training and the social norms that dictate that we must keep our thoughts to ourselves. She also had to stop her own abusive behaviors of silence and then lashing out.

Six months later Sarah came back to see me. She hadn't been able to keep the boundaries with her boyfriend at this point, yet wasn't ready to end the relationship. She was too afraid of his violence to just walk out. Understandably, she was depressed again. She had been re-traumatized by her own inability to leave the relationship when the abuse continued. A year later, she did leave the man, got a restraining order to protect herself, and returned for more sessions to clear the trauma she experienced by staying in the relationship during that year.

William: Changing old habits

We traumatize ourselves by repeating old habits. We become accustomed to our patterns and we repeat them because it is easier than trying new things that feel uncomfortable.

An example of creating that which we are attempting to change is William, who felt that people didn't listen to him. We did quite a bit of clearing regarding his issues of being heard. As a child, his view was that he was not heard or respected, and never (in his memory) were his thoughts or feelings solicited. He assumed that others did not value him or his input.

- People don't hear me.
- They don't want to listen to me.
- They don't care about what I say.
- I won't be heard no matter what I do.
- People don't value what I have to say.

How Behavioral Change Works in the CLEAR Process

After clearing these issues, William still felt that others weren't really listening to him. I asked him to examine his behavior—did he talk more than was necessary? Did others get tired of listening to him? Or when he talked, did he speak of irrelevant or unimportant things? The answer was yes to all of these questions. William realized that he was alienating people with his communication, and did need to change his behavior. He committed to speaking only when necessary, and only about important things. Within a few months, Will felt that things had shifted and people were listening; he was feeling heard for the first time in his life.

David: Re-traumatizing ourselves with our own behavior

It is important to examine our behaviors for negative patterns that could re-traumatize us. Once we identify problematic behavior, it is equally vital to find an alternative positive behavior. When the new behavior is simple, there is a much better chance that we will be successful. If we say or do something 30 times, there is a good probability that it will become a new habit. David's example is this kind of behavioral change.

At 38, David was hardworking and successful in his business. All his life he had been analytical and very reserved emotionally. He came to me because he was losing weight, wasn't digesting food properly, felt anxious and couldn't sleep at night. He saw me three times to clear trauma related to a fear of dying that began when his father died. Within two weeks he was relatively free of anxiety, sleeping normally and feeling well physically.

Once he felt physically better, he acknowledged that he wanted to act differently with his children and wife. Where he had been very critical and judgmental of the people around him, he now wanted to show them more love and warmth. In order to practice the new behavior, we decided he would give each child and his wife positive feedback on something they did at least once a week—and he would give each of them a hug once a day. He would make a concerted effort to reduce his judgmental statements, asking them to remind him when he slipped. And at work he would find something good to say about someone at least once every day. David has practiced these few behaviors and has gradually changed his relationship with his children, his wife, and his colleagues.

• • •

We also re-traumatize the body when we treat *ourselves* in a way that reflects our past treatment. If I talk negatively to myself, for example, saying, "I can't believe I am so stupid," instead of having compassion for the predicament in which I find myself, this is probably reminiscent of the ways I was treated in the past. Treating ourselves badly after clearing trauma eventually causes more trauma that needs to be cleared. The important practice of self-love is discussed more fully in Appendix B, "Understanding Love and Fear."

Even though the energy therapies are powerful tools to create change, there are times when behavioral therapy is also necessary to support the process. Clients often benefit from suggestions on how to change their behavior, particularly when they don't see the origins of a particular pattern. They may also need support and follow-up on the changes they want to create in their lives. This is essential, as old behaviors and emotions, such as being self-critical, unreasonably angry or continually fighting, can re-traumatize us.

HOW TO SECTION

In this section I describe how to heal trauma using CLEAR by identifying the issue, clearing blocking beliefs, employing muscle testing, and working with the acupressure points. Diagrams, flow charts and lists accompany the descriptions. In addition, I have provided a step-by-step guide through the process of healing.

Know that in using CLEAR, you cannot hurt yourself or the person on whom you are working. You will not make anything worse if you make a mistake or forget a step. The trauma may not fully clear, but you won't damage the person or yourself.

CHAPTER 6
Using Muscle Testing

Muscle testing makes this process clear and specific by identifying the particular issue to work on. It indicates which points are necessary to clear the issue. We also use muscle testing to ensure the issue is clear; if the issue is not clear, muscle testing helps us to figure out why. Perhaps there are blocking beliefs preventing the clearing, or there may be other points that need to be worked with before this particular point is clear. Muscle testing makes this obvious with a few simple steps.

Muscle testing others

In order to use muscle testing with energy therapies, I ask the person being tested to hold firm in a particular position while making a statement related to the issue. Usually, the person holds an arm out in front of her body, parallel to the floor. This position is easier on the shoulder than holding it out to the side and parallel to the floor.

I ask the person to hold her arm in that position or to resist me pushing her arm down. If she can hold the position, then the issue being tested is strong or the answer is a "yes." If she cannot hold the position, then there is a weakness; the answer is "no." For example, I want to see if we need to clear the issue of "I am stupid." I ask the client to hold out her arm and say, "I should

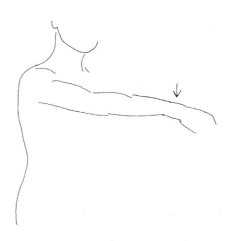

Muscle Testing

clear, 'I am stupid.'" If, when I test her arm, it holds firm, that means, "Yes, we need to clear this issue." Then I might ask the client to say, "I should begin by clearing blocking beliefs regarding this issue." Again, if the arm holds firm, that indicates a yes, and we begin by clearing blocking beliefs.

Some people get their yes's and no's reversed. If this occurs, just retrain your mind or the client's mind by saying that "a yes is when the arm or finger stays firm, a no is when it is weak." Because people can get reversed, it is a good idea to begin the process by asking the person (or yourself) to "show me a yes" and then test. You should get a strong response. Then ask the person to "show me a no" and test again. You should get a weak response.

Self-testing

It is also possible to use muscle testing techniques on yourself. To do this, make a statement to yourself while attempting to hold the thumb and index finger together in an "O" shape, and pulling another finger from the other hand through those fingers. If the finger doesn't go through then the answer is a "yes." If it does go through, it is a "no." Or you can hold one index finger out straight and attempt to push it down with your middle finger of the same hand. A final method for self-testing is to stand up and close your eyes. Say "no" and see which way your body leans (usually back) and then say "yes" and see which way your body leans (usually forward).

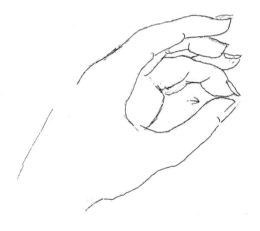

Self-testing

The best method for self-testing is the one that feels most comfortable to you. Some people have difficulty testing themselves. Don't feel that you are a failure if this is the case, just practice a bit more. If you still feel uncomfortable with it, then teach the process to another person and ask him to test for you. Or clear your blocking beliefs about being able to muscle test yourself, such as, "I don't think this will work, I can't test myself," or "I am afraid I will control the results," or "I want it to turn out a certain way." And then try muscle testing yourself again.

Creating statements to use in muscle testing

The way you phrase a question or statement may determine the outcome of muscle testing, so make sure that what you say is what you want to test. If the results are confusing, first ask if this is a valid question or statement you are testing and muscle test that. If the response is "no," try wording the question in a different way. If you are testing someone and you continually get a "no" or weak response, then start by doing a cure for a "general reversal" as described below.

CHAPTER 7
The Steps in the CLEAR Process

In each CLEAR session, we work through six steps from identifying the issue to clearing blocking beliefs related to the issue, and finally clearing the trauma and its origins. Naturally, each client's process will be slightly different, but the process is flexible and open enough to incorporate those differences.

A note about the impact of working with people

Students often ask me how I "protect myself" from other people's energy when I work with clients. I used to worry about picking up another's negative energy; however, I now believe that if I am fully present to my feelings and what arises in my own body as I work, that I won't take on anything unwanted. I will explain this more fully in the section on trauma.

Sometimes as I work with a client I realize that I may have my own issue to clear that is related to their topic. I simply make a mental or literal note about the issue, and later muscle test myself on it. If there is something to work on, I find some time when I won't be disturbed and clear it.

To create a tone of relaxation and respect, I light a candle before each session. As I begin working, I face the client, and check in with myself to make sure that I am fully in my body. I become aware of how I feel and what I am thinking. Periodically during the session, I check in with myself to make sure that I am present, in my body, and paying attention to *my* reactions, thoughts and feelings. I simply allow my responses to exist without judgment. If I am not in my body, I am not fully present and in relationship with the other person. Being present with yourself and the individual with whom you are working models how he can be present with himself, which speeds healing.

Step 1: Identifying the issue

NOTE: I describe this process from the perspective of working with a client, but you can easily use the process on yourself if you feel comfortable muscle testing yourself. Just replace "yourself" where you see references to "the client."

The first step in working with a client, is understanding the issue on which she wants to work. I may ask her why she came, what it is that she sees as the issue. In addition, I may inquire about what she wants; what, for example, would her life look like if the issue were healed. These questions often help clients see where they are blocked. I listen to what she says and how she says it and make some notes about what sound like blocking beliefs and traumas. Let's say, for example, that the issue is around work and financial success. I may write something like, "I can't be financially successful," or "I can't be a success in my work life." Next, I ask the client what beliefs she thinks may be associated with this issue, such as "I am not smart enough," or "I don't think I can be successful." You can also suggest beliefs that may be contributing to the issue, such as "I don't deserve to be happy," or "If I am successful then others will expect more of me." For more ideas regarding blocking beliefs, review the lists of blocking such beliefs throughout the book and in appendix C.

In the list below, you'll see some basic blocking beliefs that I test and clear early on, as their existence can prevent clearing of other issues.

- Energy therapies can help me/energy therapies can't help me.
- I want to live/I want to die.
- I want to be here in this body/I don't want to be here in this body.
- I can't live with my pain/I can live with my pain.
- Life is too difficult, I don't want to be here/I want to be here.
- I am deserving/I am not deserving.
- Life is hard/I enjoy living.
- I can trust myself/I can't trust myself.
- I can trust others/I can't trust others.
- I am safe/I am not safe.
- If only I could do something differently/be different, they would like me/love me.
- I am worthy/I am not worthy.
- I have to be better than others to get love.

The Steps in the CLEAR Process

- I cannot compare with others, so I will never get love.
- I have to be better than others to be successful.
- I don't have what it takes, so I won't be successful.

If you get a negative muscle test response (where the arm goes weak on the positive statement) then you need to clear it. If you get a positive muscle test (where the arm holds firm on the negative statement) then you need to clear it.

It is often a good idea to test for both negative belief and positive beliefs. For example with the beliefs, "I love myself" and "I hate myself," I may find that the client does not hate herself, but she doesn't love herself either. In this instance, the client needs to clear the belief, "I don't love myself" and probably needs to check others like "I'm not loveable," and "If I love myself, others won't like me." Often beliefs like these have trauma associated with them; that trauma also needs to be cleared using the acupressure points.

Step 2: Reversals

During muscle testing, be sure to check for reversals, which means that the body is somehow not registering correctly. Reversals can result from stress, exhaustion, dehydration, confusion, or resistance to feeling emotions associated with the trauma, all of which can disturb the body's energy field.

To test for general reversal:

Ask the person to hold her arm out in front of her. It should be parallel to the floor and directly in front of her shoulder. Ask her to hold firm when you say something like "be aware" or "notice." We don't say to "resist" the pressure because that may plant that thought in her head. Test by saying "notice," and pushing down on the person's wrist. The hand should hold firm.

Next, have the client put her other hand (the one you are not using to test) over the top of her head, palm down. Say "notice" and test the arm in front of her. Again, you should have a strong response. Have the client turn her hand over on top of her head so that the palm is facing the ceiling and test again by asking her to "notice" and pushing down on the wrist. The hand should test weak or you should feel a "give" in her resistance. This is because the hand turned over like this creates a negative charge, much like magnets

Change Works with CLEAR

do when you reverse them. Now tell the client that a strong response means a "yes" and a weak response indicates a "no." Ask her to say, "yes, yes, yes" and test again. You should have a strong response.

If any of these steps don't work, then the person is reversed and you need to do a "cure" using the acupressure points. First, try having the client rub her sore spots (above the breast, refer to illustration below), and say, "I love and accept myself, honor and respect myself with all of my problems and limitations, and I am present in my body." And test again.

If that doesn't work, then have the client try the following procedure:
- Cross the left foot over the right;
- Ask her to put her left hand on her right leg and cross the right hand over the left, placing her right hand on her left leg;
- Finally, have her put her tongue on the roof of her mouth just behind the teeth and breath normally for a few seconds.

This should clear the reversal and the person will then have normal muscle testing results. If not, check to see if there are blocking beliefs that may be impacting the muscle testing such as "I don't want to clear this," or "I don't want to feel the feelings associated with this."

Step 3: Muscle testing

Use muscle testing to determine whether you should start by clearing the person's blocking beliefs. Follow the process described below in the "Flow Chart or Outline." The next steps depend upon whether you are starting the process by clearing blocking beliefs using the acupressure points.

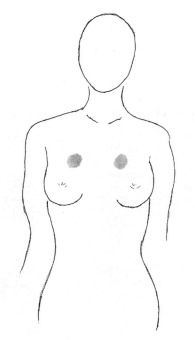

Sore Spots

Flow Chart

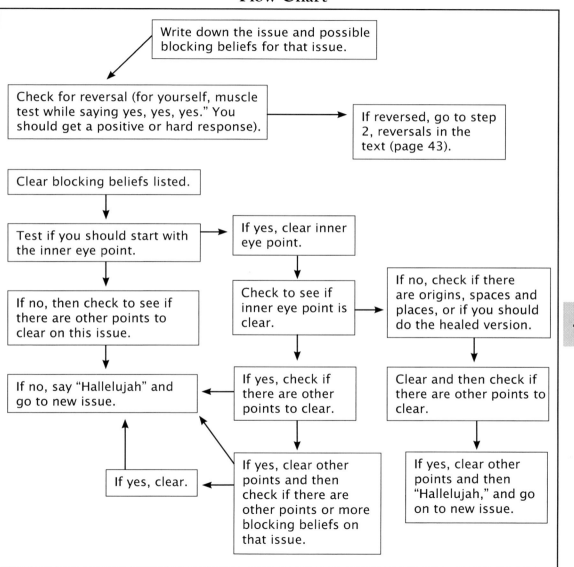

Change Works with CLEAR

Outline for clearing
1. Write down the issue and possible blocking beliefs for that issue.
2. Check for reversal. (Muscle test while saying "yes, yes, yes." You should get a positive or firm response.)
3. Clear each of the blocking beliefs you have written down in your initial discussion using the statement:

    "Even though I believe…(list the beliefs here)… I love and accept myself, I forgive myself for thinking these things, I forgive anyone who impacted me in thinking these things, and I am present in my body."

    After saying the list and repeating this statement, I ask the client to take a deep breath. NOTE: If you have difficulty with this statement, or you think your client would have difficulty with this statement, change it so that you and your client are comfortable. For example, you might say, "even though I believe_____, I love and accept myself" or "Even though I believe_____, I am present in my body."
4. Ask the client if there were sentences that had a particular "charge" to them as she cleared the beliefs.
5. Test to see if there are points to clear on the "charged" issue. If yes, test to see if the first point to clear is the inner eye point. If yes, then begin by clearing this point.

    If not, muscle test to see if there are other points to clear. If yes, refer to your sheet with the acupressure points and test each point on the list, stopping and clearing when you get to a point that needs to be cleared. If no, go on to see if there are other points or blocking beliefs to clear.
6. When you have cleared a particular point, muscle test to ensure that point is clear. If the point is clear, then test to see if there are other points to clear. If the point is not clear, then muscle test if the next step is to "do the point again." If yes, repeat the point. If no, ask if there are other steps to clear on this point (the origins, spaces and places, or healed version which are explained below). If no, ask if there are other points to clear at this time. If yes, test to see which point to do next and then clear that point. When you complete the clearing process, again check to see if that point is clear, and then again check to see if there are other points to clear on this issue.

The Steps in the CLEAR Process

7. Say something to celebrate that the issue is clear. This is to acknowledge the freeing of the issue from the system. I often say, "Yes!" or "Hallelujah!"

Step 4: Clearing blocking beliefs

In CLEAR, we release blocking beliefs by working with two points on the chest. To clear a blocking belief, I say the **statement** below and ask the client to repeat after me, while she rubs her sore spots. The sore spots are on the chest above the pectoral muscles and below the collarbone directly above the breasts (see picture on page 44). You do not need to rub them hard. A light circular touch is fine. You will make yourself sore if you rub too hard. You can clear more than one belief at a time.

For example, you could say:

> "**Even though I think I am not smart enough, and I don't deserve to be successful, and I don't want to be successful, and I am afraid of the responsibility I will have if I am successful…I love and accept myself, I forgive myself for thinking these things, I forgive anyone who impacted me in thinking these things, and I am present in my body.**"

Then take a deep breath.

NOTE: It may seem counter-intuitive to say the blocking belief in its negative form (such as, "Even though I don't love myself…"). However, by stating it this way we are raising the issue in your system, then rubbing the sore points clears it. Don't worry about putting it into one's system by making this statement. We are simply accepting that this belief is there and loving ourselves anyway. Ironically, this process clears the belief. If there is related trauma this process may be more complicated and you will need to clear one or more acupressure points in addition to the beliefs.

Muscle testing and clearing blocking beliefs may seem repetitive, but it is important to follow the process if you want to clear issues completely. It won't hurt the person with whom you are working if you forget a step or make a mistake, but it may make the process longer, and the trauma may not completely clear. Also, people say that it is helpful to hear the list of blocking beliefs as you clear them because they get to hear what they just said.

Step 5: Clearing the points

After clearing blocking beliefs, muscle test to see if there are points to clear. If there are, ask if you should start by clearing the inner eye point. If yes, begin by clearing this point. If not, then ask if there are other points to clear. If yes, refer to your list of acupressure points, test each one, stopping and clearing when you get to a point that needs it.

For most points, the client should lightly touch, rub or tap the specified point. For the inner eye point, use the following pose, which was taught to me by Tapas Fleming. The client rests her thumb and ring finger just above her tear ducts, and *lightly* pinches the bridge of her nose. She places the middle finger in between and just above the eyebrows. And then the other hand is placed on the back of your head with the thumb at the base of the head.

Put your attention on the issue, whatever it is. Remain in the position until you feel a release, a sigh, or you experience a sense that you are finished. Many people feel "lighter" when the issue is clear, or nothing further comes up.

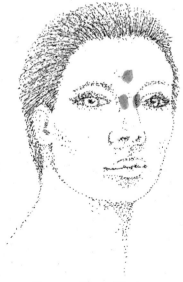

Inner Eye Point

When I work with clients, I ask them to talk to me as they clear a point if they are comfortable doing so. As they speak, I listen very carefully and take notes regarding possible blocking beliefs and other traumas related to the issue. When they are done with that point, we clear blocking beliefs that I noted as I listened to them talk.

For instance, while Sue discusses moving into a career she wants, we realize that she doesn't feel secure because she never felt wanted. We test to see if that issue needs to be cleared. The muscle testing indicates a yes, and we start with the inner eye point. While Sue is clearing the issue, "I am not wanted" she says, "My mother never wanted me, and she wanted to end the pregnancy;

she doesn't like me, and she thinks I am annoying." I write down each of those statements and then clear them as blocking beliefs using the sore points before I test whether the inner eye point is clear.

Focus when clearing

While a client is working, focusing on her body helps to reprocess the trauma. Focus on the origins of the problem helps to stimulate and then clear the trauma. Focus on the healed version of an issue to helps her to integrate new behavior. Below I describe these areas of concentration in detail.

The body

During a session, a client may experience a physical sensation while she is touching a point; this is normal and common. It may be something specific like a headache or nausea or more vague and dispersed like tension. If this occurs, I have the client put her attention on that sensation. I ask her if there is any other information in the feeling. The sensation may shift to another feeling or simply go away. If a feeling doesn't arise naturally, I often ask the client if she feels anything in her body. If she feels something in her heart, for example, I say, "Put your attention there and see if there are any sensations or other information in that place." Often she has an important insight or makes an interesting connection. This essential element provides a space for the client to feel her body and to accept the feeling in it. It stops her resistance to the sensation and it allows her to feel something difficult: she doesn't have to run from what has been a negative experience in the past. It is a powerful way for the body to acknowledge the feeling and then let it go.

Origins

When muscle testing indicates that an issue is not clear, check to see if there are "origins" related to it. Origins may be anything in a person's life that may be impacting this issue. They may be specific incidents from her own past or from her parents' lives, for example. In either case, the client focuses on the origin issue while she holds the acupressure points. It can even be something from a past life (if you believe in past lives) that relates to this issue. While the client touches the point being cleared, she puts her attention on whatever the origins are, even if she doesn't know what they are. Sometimes the client has no memory of the origins, but the process clears them anyway. She should remain in the position until she feels a release, or until she feels done with the origins. And again, muscle test to make sure the origins are clear. If they aren't, you will want to do the point again, perhaps focusing on different times in the client's life such as infancy, childhood, adolescence, or early adulthood.

Healed version

Often, clients find it very helpful to focus on the healed version of the issue. That is, what will she feel like when this trauma is no longer stuck in her body. Think of this as the opposite of the negative emotions we associate with the trauma. I make statements and ask questions such as the following to help the client understand how to envision the healed version: Focus on what you feel like without this trauma. What you are doing differently? How do you feel? What people are saying to you? How are you interacting with people?

Experiencing the healed state allows the person to feel the balance of the positive state while she clears a difficult issue. In this experience, she integrates a new way of being, bringing it in to her body at an energetic and cellular level, and providing access to it later.

For some clients, focusing on new ways of being may cause more blocking beliefs to arise about why this state couldn't occur. Usually, it is enough to take the client through the experience of the healed version once, and the point or points you use to do this can vary. Muscle test to see which point should be touched in order to instill the healed version. Next, touch the point while you have the client put her attention on what she looks like, feels like and acts like without this issue or trauma in her life. Ask her to imagine herself as fully healed from the issue on which she is working.

For example, if Sue is working on the issue of her career, she might focus on herself being successful in something she loves. She lets herself feel that in her body, how she feels in the world when she is in this healed place, and the kinds of things she is doing. If she experiences blocking beliefs about why she can't get what she wants, then we need to clear them. If she clearly experiences the new situation, then she feels that in her body and fills up with that feeling. She holds the point until she feels "full" or until she feels complete

The Steps in the CLEAR Process

with the experience. At the end of this healed version process, we muscle test to make sure that the healed version in that point is clear.

When you believe you are finished clearing a particular point, muscle test to ensure that point is clear. If it is, then test to see if there are other points to clear on that issue and move on to clearing those points. If the point is not clear, then muscle test whether you should "do it again." If yes, repeat the point. If you shouldn't do it again, ask if you should work on the origins, the body, or the healed version. Again, muscle test to see if that point is clear, and then again, check to see if there are other points to clear on this issue.

Step 6: Blocking beliefs on the issue

Blocking beliefs about an issue may create confusing results as you work through this process. Let's say, for example, a client doesn't feel it is safe to clear an issue and/or she doesn't want to work on it. If this is the case, you may not be able to clear a point, or may get confusing results about being done with the issue. For example, you might muscle test, "There are other points to clear on this issue," and get a "yes." Then you may get a "no" when you muscle test, "we should clear this now." In this case you may either ask the client what she thinks is impacting the situation, or rely on your own intuition. With either option, use muscle testing to check the ideas.

The following common beliefs may impact the clearing of an issue. When an issue won't clear or you get conflicting results from muscle testing, I recommend that you check these and then clear the ones that exist.

- Energy therapies can/can't work for me.
- This process is too simple—it can't work.
- This process is dumb; I don't like it.
- Energy therapies will never clear my issues.
- I want to/don't want to clear my trauma.
- It is safe/isn't safe to clear my trauma.
- It is safe/isn't safe to clear this issue.
- I don't want to clear this issue.
- I want to/don't want to work on this issue.
- I don't want to remember those feelings.

- If I clear this issue, I won't remember what I need to, to stay safe/to keep others safe.
- I don't deserve to clear this issue.
- I'll lose my identity if I clear this issue.
- It's not possible to clear it.
- I'll be confused if I clear it.
- I'll be hurt if I clear it.
- I may hurt others if I clear it.
- I am not ready, willing or able to clear it.

Emotions and blocking beliefs

Energy therapies do not rid us of our emotions or our difficulties in life, as I explained earlier. Emotions hold an important place in our lives and are necessary for our healing; however, our culture often teaches us to subdue and avoid these feelings. Boys may learn not to cry while girls are taught that they shouldn't be angry. When our parents try to control us by stopping our feelings we learn that emotions are inappropriate, negative and bad. Yet feeling sad is a natural, indeed healthy emotion—as is anger. When we stifle our emotions we traumatize ourselves because we are inhibiting a natural physical process.

In working with CLEAR it is important that we free negative beliefs about emotions. In this process we learn to feel our emotions, understand where they come from and what they mean to us. They exist for a reason. If we can be present with our emotions, we understand when they are connected to past events or informing us of critical information.

For example, I may feel angry and not understand why. If I sit with the feeling, it may become clear that I am angry because my husband hasn't heard something that I have been trying to tell him for a few days. Upon further examination, I may find that I never felt heard in my family. My ability to be present with these feelings allows me to see that I need to find a way to make myself heard with my husband, and I may also need to do some energy therapy work on my past issue of not being heard.

In the past, our emotions may have meant we were in danger of being hurt, having love taken away from us, or of losing control. Naturally, we don't want these outcomes, so we try to block emotion and consequently develop blocking beliefs about our emotions. To allow the natural process of being with our emotions, it is helpful to clear blocking beliefs

Addendum to go after **step 6** on page 52, and before "**Emotions and blocking beliefs**."

Bi-lateral stimulation
If you muscle test that there is something to clear but it is not blocking beliefs or acupressure points, bi-lateral stimulation might be necessary. You may also use this process if you want to quickly attenuate problematic emotions in a difficult situation (for example, for yourself during a difficult meeting or with a client when emotions get overwhelming).

Different names for this technique are used by different practitioners. I learned it as "bi-lateral stimulation." Francine Shapiro, calls it EMDR (a fairly well-known and well-researched technique used in the psychological community). Others in the energy psychology community utilize a technique called the "butterfly hug." The theory about why this process works is that the trauma is stuck on one side of the body/brain and stimulating alternating sides of the body while thinking of the situation frees it up.

This process is explained as though you were going to do it for yourself, though you may also ask your client to do the process on herself. Muscle test if bi-lateral stimulation is the next step. If so, do the following (you can also do this without muscle testing to ease your feelings in a difficult situation):

Think about the situation. Bring up any feelings you have and check-in regarding how your body feels (e.g., are you tense anywhere, do you have butterflies, feel nauseated, have pain anywhere?). Cross your arms over one another and while continuing to think about the feelings/situation alternately tap on your biceps with your hands—right, left, right left, continuing until you feel done. If crossing one arm over the other doesn't feel comfortable or is too constricting, rest your left hand on your left leg and your right hand on your right leg and alternately tap on your thighs, tap right, tap left, tap right, tap left, until you feel done. When finished, muscle test to make sure it is clear. If it is not, muscle test if you should do bi-lateral stimulation again. If yes, do that. If not, then check to see if there are acupressure points or blocking beliefs to clear on the issue.

The Steps in the CLEAR Process

about accepting and feeling emotions. The ones listed below are common. Add to the list any beliefs you have regarding your own experience with emotions.

- If I accept these emotions, I won't be safe.
- I don't want to feel my feelings.
- It's not good to feel my feelings.
- It's not safe to feel my feelings.
- It is too difficult to feel this way.
- I don't want to feel this way.
- If I accept/allow these feelings, I'll get stuck there.
- If I accept/allow these feelings, they'll take me over/I'll lose control.
- I don't want to accept my feelings.
- I need to resist feeling bad.
- If I feel my feelings, I will be unhappy.*
- Increased awareness means I will be less happy, so I don't want to be aware.*
- I don't like feeling bad.
- It's not good to feel bad (sad, terror, fear, anger, anxiety, pain).
- I shouldn't feel bad (sad, terror, fear, anger, anxiety, pain).
- I'll bring others down if I feel bad.
- I don't want to feel anger.
- I don't like being angry.
- Anger is a bad emotion.
- I won't be loved if I am sad/angry/too happy.

Obviously, there may also be trauma associated with these beliefs, so muscle test to see if each one is clear after clearing them as a group using the sore points. If they are not clear, then check to see if there are points to clear on each one.

When we feel upset, it may be helpful to view the situation as an opportunity to check for and clear trauma and blocking beliefs. This is one way to muster positive feelings toward our negative emotions. It is also useful to think about the fact that we are honoring

---

*Thanks to Derrick Jensen for the germs of these ideas.

Change Works with CLEAR

(or loving or being compassionate to) ourselves when we fully accept our feelings, which allows us to be fully present in the here and now. If we resist the present, then we are not completely in the present and do not have access to our full intelligence and our spiritual connection. Moreover, in this state we don't have to ability to fully connect with others.

This chapter led you step by step through the CLEAR process. Hopefully, you have a sense now of how to clear your trauma. In Chapter 8, I will review the acupressure points—where they are located on the body and the emotions to which they are connected.

CHAPTER 8
Learning the Acupressure Points

This chapter lists the fifteen acupressure points we use in this therapeutic practice. The points are some of the same ones used in traditional acupuncture. Each acupressure point is associated with particular emotions (see table below). During the clearing process a client often feels the emotion associated with a particular point she is holding even when she doesn't know about the relationship between the two. For example, she might be touching the outer eye point, and say, "Wow, I feel really angry." She may be stimulating the chin point and say, "I am feeling shame about this." Or she may tell a story that indicates the shame she felt regarding the issue on which we are working. This phenomenon supports the notion that the points are important in clearing the issue. If holding the points brings up feelings associated with the trauma, then we can clear those emotions that have been stuck in the system regarding that issue.

As you work through a session, muscle test each point to see which ones you need to clear on a specific issue. Start with the inner eye point and go down the list. Begin by saying, "There are points on this issue to clear." If the muscle testing results indicate a yes, then say, "We should start with the inner eye point." If the result is a "yes," then clear that point. When that point is clear, test to see if there are other points to clear. If you get a "no," then this issue is clear. If you get a "yes," then test the next point and continue this way down the list. Some of the points may be tender when you touch them particularly the under arm point, the collarbone point and what are referred to as the "sore points" since they are often tender to the touch.

In rare cases, the only points involved are the sore points. In this case the person only has blocking beliefs around the issue, but no underlying trauma. You clear the beliefs by rubbing the sore points and saying the beliefs associated with them.

Point	Location	Emotion
Inner eye	Place the thumb and ring finger in the pit of the eye and the middle finger in the middle of the forehead. Then lightly squeeze the bridge of the nose.	Trauma, frustration, fear, impatience, restlessness
Under eye	Directly under the iris on the edge of the bone, find the little "divot" or dent there.	Deprivation, disgust, bitterness, disappointment
Outer eye	Place the finger on the bone on the outside corner of the eye, so that the finger is almost pokes the eyeball.	Rage, loss of power
Under nose	Place two fingers just under the nose above the upper lip.	Powerlessness, embarrassment
Chin	Place two fingers under the lip on the chin.	Shame, defectiveness, undeserving
Collarbone	Place index fingers directly below each point of the collar bone in the indentation on each side.	Indecision, anxiety, cowardice, wanting to punish
Rib	In a straight line about 2 inches down from the nipple, under the breast on the rib.	Anger, unhappiness, resentment
Underarm	About 4 inches below the armpit, or where the bra strap would be for women.	Future anxiety, worry
Thumb	Inner side of the thumb (when the hand is palm down and the thumb is pointing toward the body). The finger pressing on the point presses against the side and bottom of the thumbnail.	Grief, intolerance, scorn, prejudice

Learning the Acupressure Points

Point	Location	Emotion
Index finger	Inner side of the index finger (when the hand is palm down and the thumb is pointed toward the body). The finger pressing on the point presses on the side and bottom of the index finger nail.	Forgiveness, guilt, unable to let negatives go
Middle finger	Inner side of the finger on the side and bottom of the nail.	Jealousy, regret, sexual tension, stubbornness
Baby/little finger	Inner side of the finger on the side and bottom of the nail.	Anger (specific)
Side of hand	Make a fist and find the crease along the side (you need not have your hand in a fist when you press on the point).	Vulnerable, sadness, sorrow
Gamut point	On the hand in between the little finger tendon and the ring finger tendon, place three fingers of the other hand.	Depression, sadness, hopeless, muddled, grief, despair, loneliness, unhappiness
Sore spots	On the chest above the pectoral muscles and below the collarbone directly above the breasts.	Used to clear blocking beliefs

Change Works with CLEAR

Inner Eye Point

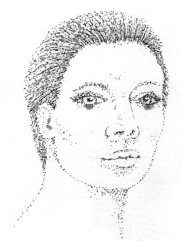

Under Eye Point

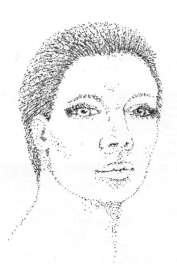

Outer Eye Point

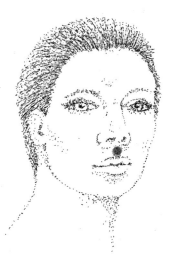

Under Nose

Learning the Acupressure Points

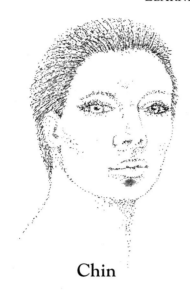

Chin

Collarbone

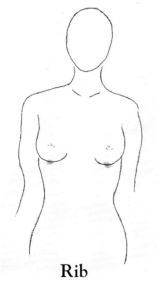

Rib

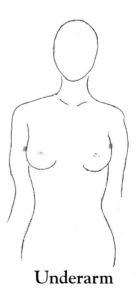

Underarm

Change Works with CLEAR

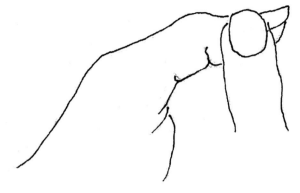

Thumb

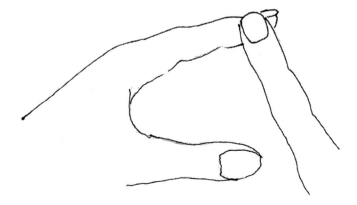

Index Point

Sore Spots

CHAPTER 9
Sample Session

In the following sample session, I offer ideas about tracking and clearing issues as you work on yourself or with a client. This demonstrates the way to burrow into an issue, and generate a list of blocking beliefs and issues as you work.

After I invite Karen into the office we sit and talk for a while about how she is doing. This is her second session. I ask her if she noticed any difference between the last session where we worked on the beliefs and traumas relating to "I am depressed," and how she feels now. She reports feeling somewhat better, a little lighter and a bit more motivated. "It isn't as difficult to get up in the morning," she says.

Moving from her progress report into her present experience, she reports that a lot of the time she was fine and even felt happy, but there were times when she felt pretty alone and isolated as if she doesn't have anyone to talk to, and she also feels trapped in her life. I ask her what it feels like to be trapped, "Like I'm stuck," she says. She wants to do something differently but doesn't know what to do.

I write down the following notes as she talks. I keep notes like these for all clients so that I can track the issues and blocking beliefs they work on. An arrow pointing left (◀) indicates that I want to check this for trauma; an arrow pointing right (▶) means this is or could be a blocking belief. Two arrows (◀ ▶) means it could be both.

- ◀ ▶ I am alone and isolated.
- ◀ ▶ I don't have anyone to talk to.
- ◀ ▶ I feel trapped.
- ◀ ▶ *No one is/was there for me* [My extrapolations are italicized].
- ◀ ▶ *No one will help me.*

- ◀ ▶ *I am afraid.*
- ▶ There is nothing I can do.
- ▶ I don't know what to do to change my situation.
- ▶ *I don't know if I can change my situation.*
- ▶ *I'm not sure I want to change my situation (then I would have to interact with people).*

I ask her if this emotional experience feels familiar to her, if there were other times in her life when she felt isolated, alone and trapped. "Oh, yes, I never had anyone to talk to growing up." Karen says, "My parents didn't care and ignored me [she had 5 siblings], and my brothers were mean to me. No one listened to me; they made fun of me, and so I stayed pretty much by myself." I ask if she felt that impacted her trust in people. After thinking for a minute Karen says, "I guess. I never thought about that, but it must have."

I write:
- ◀ ▶ They don't care for me.
- ◀ ▶ They are mean to me.
- ◀ ▶ They don't listen to me.
- ◀ ▶ They make fun of me.
- ◀ ▶ *It's not safe to share my thoughts and feelings.*
- ▶ I don't want to share.
- ◀ ▶ *They don't love me.*
- ◀ ▶ *I'm not safe.*
- ▶ *I'll be hurt if I share.*
- ▶ *I'm afraid they will hurt me.*
- ◀ ▶ I don't trust them.
- ◀ ▶ People are not trustworthy.

At this point, we have more than enough to begin, so I ask if there is anything else she wants to say before we start the muscle testing. She says, "no." And so we begin. I sit on Karen's right side and start muscle testing. First, I make sure there are no reversals. I ask her to say, "yes," and test to make sure the response is firm; it is. I ask her to say "no," and confirm that her arm has a weak response. I then tell her to say, "We should start by

Sample Session

clearing blocking beliefs." The muscle test response is firm so I know we should start by doing that. Thus, we begin by clearing blocking beliefs. We go to the sore spots and she rubs while repeating the following:

> "Even though they don't care for me; they are mean to me; they don't listen to me; they make fun of me; it's not safe to share; I don't want to share; they don't love me; I'm not safe; I'll be hurt if I share; I'm afraid they will hurt me; I don't trust them; people are not trustworthy; I love and accept myself, I forgive myself for thinking these things, I forgive anyone who impacted me in thinking these things, and I am present in my body."

Throughout the course of the whole session, I ensure that each of these beliefs and traumas is clear. I don't need to check them all now—I work through them each starting from the top—but want to make sure that I do by the time we are done. If I don't, then it is a good idea to check them in the next session. There is a good chance that quite a few of these beliefs have traumas associated with them. Moreover, it can be difficult to clear all of these traumas in a single session. For that reason, I want to keep track of what is clear and what we may need to clear in the next session. Know that it is common when someone first begins the process for there to be lots of beliefs and traumas that come up. In my experience, the process of clearing goes faster the more you clear.

The first belief and possible trauma that I wrote down was: "I am alone and isolated," so I start with this one. I ask Karen to say this statement and I muscle test. Her arm holds firm, so I know there are other points to clear regarding being alone and isolated. I ask her to say, "There are points to clear on this," to make sure. When I muscle test the response is a "yes." Then I ask her to say, "I should clear the inner eye point on 'I am alone and isolated'." The response is affirmative. I show her the pose for this point and ask her to talk to me as she puts her attention on this issue. I tell her she can start with her current feelings about being alone, and then to go back in time remembering other times when she felt this way, thus getting at the origins of this experience.

Karen says that she feels alone and everything is dark. I tell her to put her attention on the darkness and see if there is any information in the darkness as she continues to hold the inner eye point. "It is scary and my heart is beating hard," she reports.

I say, "Put your attention on your heart beating and see if there is any information in that."

She says, "No one is there for me and I'm afraid no one cares."

I write down:
- ◀ ▶ No one is there for me.
- ◀ ▶ No one cares about me.

Karen says, "Now I am remembering a time when one of my brothers locked me in the closet and I was in there forever. They forgot about me." I ask her what happened. Still holding the inner eye point, Karen continues. "I gave up yelling and it was hours before someone opened the door. I think I missed dinner. I can't believe they left me in there all day! Jeez, that's like abuse."

I tell her to sit with how it felt abusive and I write down:
- ▶ I can't believe they left me in there all day.

"Now I am remembering another time," she continues, "when I was walking with my brothers in the woods and they started running and I couldn't keep up. I was all alone in the woods and I sat down and cried. After a while I realized I would have to start walking or I would be there all day. So I started walking home. I can't believe they were that mean."

I write down:
- ▶ I can't believe they were that mean.

While Karen is still holding the inner eye point I ask if there is anything else about being alone and isolated. "Yes," she says, "I am remembering when I found out that my last boyfriend was sleeping around. I felt that way then. I also couldn't believe it." I tell her to put her attention on how she felt when she found out her boyfriend was sleeping around, and ask her if there is anywhere in her body where she feels it. "Yes, in my stomach," she says. I tell her to put her attention on her stomach and see if there is other information there. She says, "Yes, I'm scared of men. I'm not even sure I want one around."

Sample Session

I write down:
- ▸ I can't believe he was sleeping around.
- ◂ ▸ I can't trust men.
- ▸ I'm not sure if I want a man around.
- ◂ ▸ *I'm not safe with men.*

I go on and ask if there is anything else about being alone and isolated. Karen says, "No, I don't think so." I tell her she can stop and ask her to go to her sore points. She rubs those points and clears by repeating after me as I read down the list of blocking beliefs I have created:

"Even though I think that no one cares about me and I can't believe they left me in there all day, and I can't believe they were that mean, and I'm not sure if I want a man around, I can't trust men, and I'm not safe with men; even though I think these things, I love and accept myself, I forgive myself for thinking these things, I forgive anyone who impacted me in thinking these things, and I am present in my body."

I then muscle test this statement: "The inner eye point on I am alone and isolated is clear." The test indicates a yes, so I ask her to say, "There are other points to clear on this issue." The result is a "yes," and so I say the next point on the list of acupressure points, the under eye point. She repeats it and I test. The answer is "yes" so I know that is the next point to work on. I show her the point and again ask her to hold the point lightly and talk to me about what comes up while she is touching that point and putting her attention on the issue.

After about a minute, she says, "It feels like my chest is vibrating." I tell her to put her

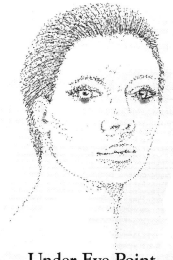

Under Eye Point

attention on that vibrating in her chest and see if there's any information there. She says, "I'm afraid and I don't want to be here." I write down:
- ◀ ▶ I'm afraid.
- ◀ ▶ I don't want to be here.

I ask her to put her attention on not wanting to be here. She cries and says, "It is so hard. It's not supposed to be this hard. Why does it have to be so hard? It doesn't seem fair."

I write down:
- ▶ It's not supposed to be this hard.
- ▶ It doesn't seem fair that it is this hard.

She stays in the pose and seems to calm down. I ask how she is doing. She says, "I feel calmer, and it is brighter—like the sun is shining outside even though I have my eyes closed."

"Good," I say. "What does that feel like?"

"It's difficult to explain," Karen responds, "kind of like things are falling into place—like I am more aligned.

I tell her she can stop now, knowing that the sensation of more light and being more aligned is a sign that the issue is clear.

I ask her to go to her sore points and repeat after me:

"Even though I'm afraid and I don't want to be here, and it's not supposed to be this hard, and it doesn't seem fair that it is this hard; even though I think these things, I love and accept myself, I forgive myself for thinking these things, I forgive anyone who impacted me in thinking these things, and I am present in my body."

I then muscle test to see if the under eye point on "I am isolated and alone" is clear. It is, so I ask if there are other points to clear on this. There are not, however, I want to go back to an issue that she said about not wanting to be here. This is a big issue and can impact other issues, so I want to make sure it is clear before we go on. I ask her to say, "I want to be here." And I test her. Her arm goes down, meaning no, she doesn't want to be here, so there are still beliefs or traumas to clear on this. I ask her to say, "There are points to clear on this," and the result is that there are. I start by testing the inner eye point. The result is a no, so I go to the outer eye point, skipping the under eye point because we were doing this point when the issue came up. The muscle testing indicates that we should clear the outer eye point next. I ask her to touch the outside edge of her eye on the bone lightly, to close her eyes, put her attention on the issue of not wanting to be here and talk to me about what comes up while she does that.

Karen says, "My parents weren't there for me. I guess they were really busy, but they never talked to me or asked how I was. They didn't protect me from my brothers or tell them that they shouldn't do what they did to me. I know my parents did what they could, but now I am feeling really angry. I don't think I should be feeling angry at them."

I write down:
▸ I don't think I should feel angry at them.
▸ I don't want to be angry.
▸ I shouldn't be angry.

I tell Karen, "It's okay to feel the anger. Just let yourself feel it, and see if it is anywhere in your body."

"Yes, it is in my upper chest and shoulders," she reports. I tell her to put her attention there and see if there is any information there for her.

"Why would anyone have kids and not want to take care of them?" she questions. "It was irresponsible for them not to be there for me! They shouldn't have had so many kids. They weren't mature enough to have kids. Wow, I can't believe I just said all of that. I know they did the best they could."

I write down:
▸ I can't believe I said all of that.

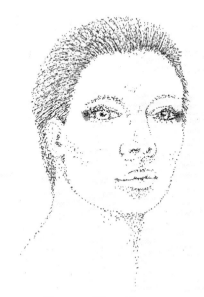

Outer Eye Point

▸ *I shouldn't feel negative feelings.*

I ask her to continue holding the outer eye point and tell her, "It is okay—it's good to feel what you feel. It is a way of honoring yourself. Let yourself feel it and see if there is other resistance to it."

She states, "No, I can see why I would be upset. It makes sense, and I can feel the shifting in my body."

"Good," I tell her, "now go back to your chest and shoulders and check in. How does it feel now?"

She reports that it feels better. I tell her she can stop and I ask her to go to her sore spots, and we clear the four beliefs she said while doing that point. Then I check to see if the outer eye point is clear on the issue, "I don't want to be here." It is, so I check to see if there are other points to clear on that. The next point that we need to clear is the chin point. I show her how to hold the point and ask her to put her attention on the issue and talk to me about what comes up.

She says, "I never wanted anyone to come over to my house. I didn't want people to see how mean my brothers were. I mean, I didn't like it there, so why would my friends? I guess I was embarrassed about my family. My best friend's parents were so loving, and I didn't want her to see how…selfish my parents were. Wow. I never thought about it that way before. I guess they were selfish."

I write down:
▸ I don't want people coming over to my house.
▸ I don't think they'll like it here.

I ask her how that feels that her parents were selfish. "It's sad," she states. "I mean, it's sad for me; it's sad for them. It's just sad."

"Yes, it is sad," I tell her. "Let yourself just feel the sadness, and see if there is anything else about this issue."

"Well, just that I feel bad for them," she says, "like they were missing out on life. I guess that's it."

I tell her she can stop doing the chin point and ask her to go to her sore points to clear the two beliefs that came up. Then I ask her how she is doing. She lets me know that she is fine, sort of surprised by what is coming up, but that she feels good. I check to make sure the chin point is clear on the issue of not wanting to be here. It is not clear. We muscle test, "I should do the point again and focus on origins." The answer is no, so we test, "We should do the point again and focus on places in the body." The answer is a yes. We go to the chin point again and focus on "I don't want to be here" and see if there is any place in her body where she feels anything.

"Yes, in my throat," Karen reports. I tell her to put her attention on her throat and see what information is there. She says, "Oh, I feel like throwing up." I tell her to stay with that feeling and see where it goes. "It just feels really yucky," she continues. "I don't like being in my house. I don't want to be here. I don't want to be with these people. I don't want them to be my family. I want to scream. I want to tell them they are all a bunch of losers."

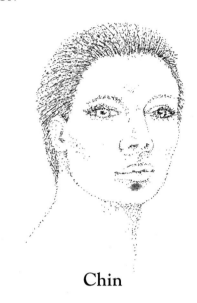

Chin

I write down:
- ▸ I don't like being in my house.
- ▸ I don't want to be here.
- ▸ I don't want to be with these people.
- ▸ I don't want them to be my family—they are losers.

Next I ask her to put her attention on wanting to scream. "I feel like I could be violent. That is scary," she reports. I tell her it is okay, everyone feels violent sometimes; it is a human thing. It is okay to feel it—we know she is not going to act on it. She is a bit shocked when she hears herself say, "I wanted them dead." She continues, "I am ashamed of myself because I had thoughts that I didn't want them to exist, and I wished that they would die in a car crash." She pauses for a while, so I ask if there is more on that. She says that there is not. I ask her to stop doing the chin point and ask how she feels. "Okay, but guilty that I have these feelings."

I write down:
- I shouldn't have those feelings.
- *I can't forgive myself for these thoughts.*

We clear the six beliefs that came up in this round and then I test to see if the chin point is clear on the issue of not wanting to be here. It isn't. We test if there are other things to clear from this point, and the answer is no. I test if there are blocking beliefs to clear. No. Then I test if there are other points to clear in order to clear the chin point. Periodically, you will find that this happens. The point you are trying to clear will not clear unless you clear other points first. Karen's muscle test indicates a "yes." I test to see if we need to clear the index finger point next since that is the point for forgiveness and guilt, and I know that is the last emotion Karen was feeling was guilt. Again, the answer is yes, so I ask her to say, "I should clear this point while thinking about my guilt," which we test. The answer is yes. I ask her to put pressure on the index finger point and put her attention on her feelings of guilt and forgiving herself for feeling these things.

While holding the index finger point, she says "I guess I can see why I had those feelings. Kids need more attention than that. I mean, I don't even remember hugging anyone in my family. That's not right. I guess I thought that if something tragic happened, I might get noticed."

I write down:
- If something tragic happens, I might get noticed.
- *I want something tragic to happen.*

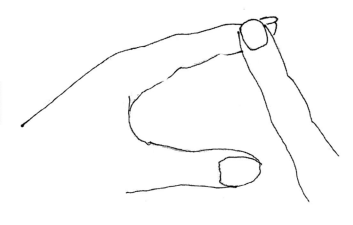

Index Point

Sample Session

She continues, "I guess I always thought it was bad to even think thoughts like that. One's mind should be more pure. If I were to be a good person, I wouldn't think thoughts like that."

I write down:
- I always thought it was bad to think thoughts like that.
- One's mind should be more pure.
- If I were a good person, I wouldn't think thoughts like that/bad thoughts.

I suggest that she continue to hold the index finger point and let herself just feel what it feels like to have thoughts about wanting her parents to die. "Well, I can see why I would," she says, "I mean I was so alone and so scared, and I was so mad at them."

I tell her that makes sense to me, too. Next I question if there is more on forgiving herself. She states, "No." And I tell her to continue holding the index finger point and say, "I forgive myself." She does, since it sounds a little tentative, I ask her to say it again. This time she says it with more conviction, so I move on. We clear the beliefs that came up while she held this point, and then I check that the index finger point is clear on guilt and forgiveness. It is. I talk to her for a minute about how it is normal for humans to have the kinds of feelings she had, and that it doesn't make her a bad person to have them—that it is only bad if one acts on those kinds of feelings. She appreciates the conversation.

At this point, I want to go back and make sure that the chin point is clear on "I don't want to be here," so we check that, and it is clear.

I now sense that Karen is tired, so I ask her how she feels. She feels good, but tired. I check to see if there is more to clear today. Yes, there is more to clear. I go back up to our initial list and start going down the list. I ask her to say, "We should clear I am trapped next." No. So we keep going down the list until we get to, "They don't care for me," which the muscle testing indicates is the one we need to work on, and then the muscle testing reveals that we need to do the inner eye point on this issue. I ask her to hold that point while she puts her attention on this issue and talks to me about what comes up.

"I can see my Dad walking in the door. He walks right past me and goes into the fridge. I am screaming inside for him to look at me, notice me, but he gets out a beer and goes to the living room. I feel devastated."

I inquire if there is a place in her body that resonates with this devastation. "Yes, there is," she reports, " in my stomach."

"Put your attention there," I say, "and see if there is more information there."

"Yes," she says. "I feel like I'm trapped. There is nothing I can do. Nowhere to go, nothing that gets me what I want." When I ask what she wants, she cries, and says, "I want him to hold me." I tell her to stay with that feeling for a minute. "Wow," she declares. "I can see this pattern in my relationships now. I want something and I scream inside, but I never say anything, and I usually end up disappointed."

I write down:
- I feel like I'm trapped.
- There is nothing I can do.
- Nowhere to go, nothing that gets me what I want.
- I shouldn't ask for what I want.
- I will end up disappointed.
- He won't give it to me.

She doesn't say anything for a bit, so I ask her to imagine what it would feel like to be cared for (this is the "Healed Version"). She says she is not sure what that would feel like. I tell her to imagine how she feels when she really loves someone or felt loved. She says, "I can do that." I suggest that she fill up her body with that feeling and then when she feels done, she can stop, which she does. We clear the above beliefs, and then I check to see if the inner eye is clear on "they don't care for me." It is, so I check to see if there are other points to clear on this. No. So I check again if there is anything else to clear now. No. I ask her how she feels. She states that she feels tired, and like that was a lot. She says she feels she made a lot of connections, and she wants some time to process all that we did. I tell her that makes sense, that it was a lot, that it is common to feel tired, and that there is more to clear, but we can do that in another session. We have worked for two hours, and that is about what most people can tolerate.

I ask her to watch for subtle shifts in how she feels and behaves. I let her know that she should feel better, but there are times when the clearing of something can start the process of other things coming up. I remind her that her coping mechanism is the same regardless of the trauma, so not to be surprised if she still has some symptoms of withdrawal or depression. She asks when she should come to see me again, and I say a week to two weeks. We schedule some time in a couple of weeks. I ask her to call if she has any questions or concerns, and ask her if she has any questions before she goes. She says, "No," so I see her out.

Karen has a fair amount of trauma from her past, so she will probably come to see me about six more times in the following few months. After that, she may come three or four times a year as needed. For example, if she lost her job and in the process of applying for new employment, realized that she is stuck because her history is filled with blocking beliefs about her ability to be successful. Or she may fall in love and realize that she has more to clear about safety and loving others. Or she may have an interaction with her boss that brings up fear, which she associates with her fear of her father and brothers.

As I work I keep track of what we have cleared and if there is anything left that wasn't cleared. I make a note to myself at the beginning of the chart if there are left over issues or beliefs that need to checked and possibly cleared in the next session. I keep all my charts in a safe place, and assure my clients that what they share with me is confidential.

APPENDIX A
The Evolution of Acupressure Point Energy Therapy

In 1996, after burning out as an organizational consultant and deciding to seek a new life-work path, I was in the midst of other difficult times with my relationship and depression. In the largest sense, powerful old patterns grasped me in a grip I couldn't seem to shake in spite of years of therapy and dedicated change work.

My dear friend Les Daroff suggested that I come to see him for Eye Movement Desensitization Reprocessing (EMDR) and Thought Field Therapy (TFT). Frankly, EMDR and TFT sounded a little "hokey" and, just too good to be true. How could any therapy work so quickly to change those issues that I had been working so hard to change for so long? Maybe the truth was that earlier, I just wasn't in enough pain to take Les up on the offer. This time, I said yes. I worked once a week for six months. In each session we did EMDR and TFT on specific issues and patterns that originated early in my life yet still impacted me in negative ways.

In the first session, we focused on my fear of being hurt. Each time we did EMDR and the issue cleared, I felt my brain do a flip, and I laughed. Les asked me how I felt about the issue, and I just laughed. Obviously, it didn't bother me any more.

At the end of each session, Les used a technique called "muscle testing" to check if the issue was clear. The result? The issue was, indeed, clear. Did this really mean, I asked him in disbelief that the issue wouldn't impact my behavior any more? He affirmed it: my system was free of this issue. I found it difficult to believe, but Les simply said, "Let's wait and see."

Imagine my joy when I discovered that day after day in situation after situation, that my defensive behavior linked to the fear of being hurt had shifted. I could examine these triggering situations much more objectively, allowing me to see that though someone else was upset, it was not necessarily about me. I didn't even have to try—I just witnessed myself being different.

In 20 years in the change business, working with individuals and groups, I had never seen anything actually remove the triggers for ineffective behavior patterns. This was the most powerful change tool I ever experienced and of course I wanted to learn to do "energy therapy" myself. It was the beginning of a journey in which I investigated many methods and approaches, all of which influenced my development of CLEAR.

I began my energy-therapy education with a relatively simple approach, Tapas Acupressure Technique (TAT) developed by Tapas Flemming. This technique, which primarily employs a major acupuncture point at the bridge of the nose, is specifically used to clear trauma. Tapas taught me about focusing on the "origins" during the healing process, that is, events from the past that may still be impacting the issue. She was also the first person who taught me that "spaces and places" are important in the healing process. Places in a person's body, for example, a sick feeling in the stomach, may connect to the trauma. In addition, it may be helpful for someone to revisit actual places in the world such as a room, a house, a quiet glade in the woods to heal the trauma.

Tapas also understood that a person's ability to imagine the "healed version" is vital in the healing process. The healed version is the alternate view of life where the trauma is no longer an issue, but just a memory without any negative impact on behavior or health. Focusing on the healed version while doing the energy therapies helps us to feel positive emotions and the potential for healing. It may also bring up those issues that are still blocking the clearing. I will always be grateful to Tapas for her contributions to my life and work.

My next educational excursion took me into Thought Field Therapy (TFT). This fairly complex process, developed in 1981 by cognitive psychologist Dr. Roger Callahan, gave me more understanding of acupressure points and their connections to emotions. TFT eliminates disturbances created by negative emotions by using key meridian points in specific sequences.

Gary Craig's Emotional Freedom Technique (EFT) is a simplified version of TFT that helped me to see that one can simplify the TFT process; therapy needn't be complex to work.

The Evolution of Acupressure Point Energy Therapy

After TFT, I moved on to Semorg Matrix, a therapeutic technique using chakras that was developed by Nahoma Asha Clinton. Clinton's method utilizes chakras as the treatment points, and assumes that there are many blocking beliefs involved in trauma. Both Les Daroff and Clinton deepened my understanding of the importance of clearing blocking beliefs in completely removing the effects of old trauma.

Eye Movement Desensitization and Reprocessing (EMDR), was developed by Francine Shapiro in 1987. This process works by having the client move his or her eyes back and forth (either following the therapist's hand movement or with a machine) while thinking of the trauma. This process also works with tactile and auditory signals, which allows clients to close their eyes during the process. EMDR is the most researched treatment utilized for Post Traumatic Stress Disorder (PTSD). Extensive research on EMDR indicates this treatment delivers significant positive changes in subjects with Post Traumatic Stress Disorder (PTSD).

Finally, I learned Peter Levine's "Somatic Experiencing" which is based on his observations of how animals react to and process trauma in the wild, and how this is different from the way that humans process of the same kind of traumatic events. Levine noted that the rational mind often prevents humans from experiencing trauma and a natural body process of trauma the way animals do, and thus, the trauma gets stuck in the body. This method convinced me of the importance of integrating feelings in the body into my practice.

Over time, in my own practice, I realized some of these processes work better for some people. For example, a client may prefer using the chakras over acupressure points. Or, for some trauma, in some clients, it is necessary to employ bilateral stimulation (a form of EMDR where you tap the client alternately on one side of the body and then on the other) creates a release. In each case, I use muscle testing to decipher the correct process for each client.

The process I explain in this book evolved over a decade, and borrows from many different methods and theories. I followed others' teachings and my own instincts in creating this system. I encourage others to make the process their own, taking what makes sense and changing it when necessary to create the most effective model they can for their own healing and healing work.

APPENDIX B
The Underlying Principles of Energy Work

There are basic principles that underlie energy therapy work as it is described in this book. You don't need to believe the principles in order for the energy therapies to work, however, you may find benefits to your healing to explore these concepts. Understanding the principles and living accordingly helps you to take charge of your life and manifest your desires. The principles arise from a combination of the study of quantum physics, chaos theory, and from psychological and spiritual practices and teachings that I have experienced.

We are all connected

Lynne McTaggart, a research journalist, wrote a book called *The Field*, which explores the concept that we are all made up of energetic charges and we are all linked through one, underlying energy field (McTaggart, 2002). Some say, "We are all one." Energy flows through us all. This energy is the difference between life and death. When we are alive, we have this energy flowing through us. When we are dead, it no longer flows through us. This is why some say that Spirit, God, or Goddess is called "The Creator." It creates us or gives us life. Many people see this energy as God or Goddess or Spirit or the "Ultimate Presence."

The wisdom of the body may lie in the wisdom of the Universe. There are many scientific studies and resulting theories that indicate that we are connected to one another and the universe through a field called the "Zero Point Field." McTaggart describes the field as the force that accounts for the stability of the atom and thus the stability of all matter. It is hypothesized by many that this field is our collective consciousness: it is what gives us access to the wisdom in the universe.

As McTaggert hypothesizes, this field is what makes distance healing, prediction, telekinesis, and other forms of extrasensory perception (ESP) possible. A number of scientists studying quantum physics and mathematics work in this area. Their studies indicate that the human mind can indeed influence chance, predict future events, and heal through prayer, shamanism, and other methods. They have also shown that individuals can successfully describe physical locations through "remote viewing," even at a great distance. Scientists have also successfully measured the electrical charges emitted from the body and shown that these charges match the locations of the Chinese acupuncture meridians.

Most of us who work with energy or who are very spiritual need no proof of this field. We know it exists and we work in a way that actually demonstrates its existence. One of the theories regarding why healing methods work is that the healer or the method transmits a coherent energy to the person needing healing. Studies of illness indicate that those with disease have lost the natural rhythm and coherent energy that exists in a healthy body. The healer or healing modality brings order to the disordered energy, thus restoring health to the person with disease. Energy therapies and acupuncture points work with the individual's energy to clear blocks and rebalance this discord, bringing the body to a healthy level of functioning.

If we see ourselves as linked to the field, then we must impact others as we heal our energetic field. As we free ourselves from our discordant energy, we help to heal others and the planet through our connection and interaction with the field. It is exciting to know that we are not only healing ourselves, but that healing radiates out to others and then others—having a healing impact perhaps beyond our wildest dreams. The scientific advances regarding the field are stimulating and hard to deny. Perhaps one day all healing will occur through energetic treatments so that operations and drugs will seem prehistoric and uncivilized. So those of you who use the field in your work, keep it up, and know there is significant scientific evidence supporting your work.

We know that when we touch another being, an exchange of electromagnetic energy from heart to brain occurs (p 160, Childre & Martin, 1999). This phenomenon is demonstrated in an experiment explained by Deepak Chopra, M.D., in *Ageless Body, Timeless Mind* (1993). In this experiment, a war veteran was hooked up to a machine, which could detect small amounts of stress in the body. He was shown pictures (such as a town being bombed), which would create a certain level of stress. When he viewed the pictures, the stress levels recorded on the machine went up markedly. The researchers then took some cells from the roof of the man's mouth and put them in a Petri dish. They took the dish into another room, and hooked the cells up to a similar machine. They showed the man the pictures again, and at the same moment that his recorded stress level increased, so did the level of the cells in the Petri dish. They then took the cells a few miles away and conducted the same experiment with the same results!

This connection can also be explained by quantum physics through a strange phenomena known as non-locality. Non-locality is demonstrated in experiments showing that when two photons are emitted from an atom, they may go off in different directions, but when one is prodded, the other twitches; when one collapses, the other collapses, no matter how far they are apart. Location ceases to exist in the quantum realm, and it is "meaningless to speak of anything as being separate from anything else" (Talbot, 1991).

The notion of non-locality and the results of Chopra's study offer a number of implications. The immediate and simplest implication is that we are more connected to knowledge and information than we think we are. There may be, for example, some legitimacy to psychics and others who know things they seemingly have no way of knowing. Many feel that non-locality is an explanation for how we know things before they happen (like knowing who is on the phone before we pick it up). Perhaps we should pay more attention to our intuitions, and encourage others to share theirs. We have access to more information than we like to think. This is not to say that we should ignore our logical thought processes, but rather to acknowledge the more subtle ideas that come in the form of intuitive hunches or gut feelings.

If we are truly this connected, then we have a responsibility to the planet and the people on the planet. Given the "butterfly effect," in which small disturbances can have large impacts on the outcome (the classic example being the flutter of a butterfly wing in the US creating a weather disturbance in Japan), it would be wise to look before we leap, and to be as aware as we can be of what we do and the impact it has. We need to align our values and vision of a greater world with how we conduct ourselves and with what we say and do to others and the environment. What we think and do impacts others, probably at levels we do not even understand. It is for this reason that we must become aware of our impact, and remember our connection.

There is enough to go around

We are smart enough and have enough resources to provide for every living thing. Remember we are all connected; what we do to others we do to ourselves. Share. Help others. Appreciate others. Be kind. Be responsible to the environment and things around you. They are you. Remember: You receive from the world what you give to the world. What you want, give away, and it will come home to you. If it doesn't, then you probably have blocking beliefs—and perhaps trauma—related to self-love, deserving or worthiness.

We are raised to think that we have to be better than others in order to receive love or be successful. This results in an attempt by people to prove that they are better than others. Somehow, if we acknowledge another's talents, we will be "less than" and miss out. The whole scenario puts us in constant competition with others. We forget that we are unique beings with unique strengths and gifts.

We compete to get ahead. We have to prove we are better and smarter than others, more powerful than others, and we have more than others. Or we give up and feel defeated because we believe we can't compete, we aren't smart enough, we don't have what it takes. These beliefs result in a vicious cycle of competition and greed and a loss of creative input from those who withdraw. They are the cause of many (if not all) wars. Religions and governments declare that they have "the way," and then they fight others to get power and to prove that they are right.

These beliefs eat away at the fabric of our communities and destroy the environment. We each need to do our part to listen to others and perhaps learn from them. And we need to clear beliefs related to the need to be better than others, so that we use one another's creativity. As a result, the world will be a healthier place for our children and their children. We should remind our children daily that they are no better than anyone else, nor are they any worse than anyone else. We are all unique, and we all have something to bring to the table. We should encourage others not to compare themselves, but to find their unique gifts and talents. Imagine what society could be like if we encouraged everyone to be the best they could be rather than competing with others!

We create our reality
> *"If you choose unconsciously, you evolve unconsciously. If you choose consciously, you evolve consciously."*
>
> Gary Zukav

Our thoughts and beliefs create our reality, and our thoughts and beliefs are a result of how we choose to perceive. If we are aware, we can choose. If we are not aware, then our thoughts basically have control over us. Given that we are aware, we can choose our state of mind. We choose our thoughts, our emotions, and our actions. Therefore, we create our reality; we are responsible for what is occurring. Remember: it is what you *be* that determines who you are, not what you do. We need to be what it is we want.

The idea that we create our reality is complicated by the fact that we live in an environment with other people and factors that co-create our world. For example, living in an area where toxic waste exists can impact one's health regardless of one's state of mind. There are factors of genetics that impact us, as in the case of some diseases or deficiencies. Moreover, other people and their actions impact us. In the holographic view of the world, everything impacts everything else, and everything that occurs is an interaction of many factors. But the main factor and often the only one we can control in this mix, is our own thought process and our ability to change or reframe our outlook. This fundamental element impacts our lives immensely. When I speak of creating reality, it is from this perspective that I speak.

We cannot create our reality if we are unconscious, and it is even more difficult if we have severe or repetitive trauma. This is because our bodies are wired to respond quickly (in the reptilian brain with the fight or flight and immobility response) to keep safe. Overcoming reactions triggered by traumas is impossible if we are unconscious, and difficult even if we are conscious. If we are unconscious, we don't even know that the reactions rule us. If we are conscious, we may try to stop the reaction, but the power of the amygdala (an almond-shaped area in the center of the brain that regulates autonomic behavior) and the resulting fear response is faster and stronger than our ability to control them. This is why the energy therapies are so important: they allow us to be free of traumas that stimulate responses that are not helpful in our lives. It is not exactly clear why the energy therapies work this way, but case studies and the practice of clearing shows us that they do, indeed clear trauma that stimulates the fight-or-flight or immobility response, thus clearing these responses from the system.

Newtonian scientists believed that they could be objective. We now know that this is no longer the case. The replicated results of experiments done by physicists indicate that electrons and photons interact constantly with their environment, changing as a result of this interaction with their surroundings. What we see is a result of what we expect to see and how we look. The observer impacts the outcome because of their expectations. Being aware of this fact encourages us to monitor and shift our negative thoughts and feelings to positive ones. One of the easiest ways to do this is through gratitude.

Thankfulness and forgiveness

Thankfulness and forgiveness facilitate contentment in life. Studies show that these emotions immediately bring the electromagnetic field into a coherent pattern (emanating from the heart), which stimulates the biological systems of the body to work in harmony (Childre and Martin, 1999). Stress and its negative effects are reduced when we are thankful. Being in the place of gratitude draws to you even more of that for which you are thankful, which in turn produces even more contentment. It is important to change the negative valance of a difficult situation to a positive in order to reduce stress. We can do this by recognizing the learnings we are receiving or may receive from the experience, and being thankful for those learnings.

Forgiveness allows us to let go. Forgiveness is more for our own peace of mind than for the benefit of the other person. When we forgive someone, we let go of our righteous anger, or our need to distance the person from us. This also reduces stress. Forgiveness is not always easy, because we may think that if we forgive the person, we accept their behavior. Or we may think that if we forgive them, our forgiveness will shift the energy of keeping them distant and allow them back into our lives—and that may feel dangerous.

Forgiveness does not mean either of those things. We can still see that the behavior was hurtful, and we can still choose not to have the person in our life.

Energy therapies can help us with forgiveness. This kind of therapy can clear the blocking beliefs and trauma associated with the issue so that we are free to forgive. When we forgive, we understand that the person who we forgive is a flawed human being, and we let go of our need to have even a small piece of anger, hate, or superiority toward them. This helps to clear our system of anything that we are attempting to push away from us (which creates trauma and stress). Practice gratitude and forgiveness daily—they heal your stress and create more contentment in life.

The importance of emotions

"I still don't know, so late in the game, how to make peace with being out of control, a condition so intrinsic to life that it seems ludicrous that I'm not wired better to accept it."

Gregg Levoy

Our emotions are barometers for how well aligned we are in our life. If we are content, we are doing well. If we are unhappy or angry, we are not doing so well. This does not mean we are always comfortable, for sometimes life lies beyond what is comfortable. Learn how to be in a place of contentment or peace even when discomfort prevails—how to contain or hold the feelings of discomfort. If we allow the discomfort to be with us, in our body, while in a state of relaxation, we prevent new trauma from forming in the body, and we prevent the strengthening of old trauma already in the system. As Steven Johnson says in his fascinating book about the brain, *Mind Wide Open*, "If your body loads up with the fight-or-flight response, the memory grows more pronounced—even if you're simply recalling events that took place in the past" (Johnson, 2004).

Our temptation is to run from uncomfortable feelings or to do something to distract ourselves from them, like eating, watching television or working. It is this act of avoiding our feelings that registers them as traumas in our system, because we don't allow the body to feel what it needs to in order to process it completely. If we accept the feelings and allow them in the body without trying to push them away or without acting out on them we can process and understand the feelings. If we try to get away from them, then we are sending a message to the system that this is dangerous, and it is likely that the memory will be stored as a trauma.

Without our emotions, we are unconscious. Learn to listen to yourself, for emotions can provide critical information regarding reality. This is not always easy, as our feelings are not always comfortable. It requires that we become comfortable within the discomfort of those feelings. This is a state of being where we are able to sit with the feeling in a state of acceptance even though there are feelings of anxiety, anger, depression or stress. It means we learn to sit with these feelings and understand what they mean—without pushing them away or denying them and without acting out on them (by doing something like yelling because of our anger or anxiety).

We allow the feelings to exist while attention is on the body and not the head. With attention on the head, the tendency is to think about the problem and try to solve it or to justify our behavior. If we put our attention on the body, we understand the origins more clearly, and we are more likely to have compassion for ourselves in the process. Being in the head when you feel something uncomfortable tends to make stress worse. Being in the body brings understanding—and often relief—to the discomfort.

Feeling our emotions is an act of kindness to the self. It is an acknowledgement that there is something going on, and it honors our process. We need to learn to have compassion for having the feelings. Ask, Why am I angry/upset/unhappy? Be willing to dig deep and be present with the feelings. Flow with the essence of who we are and be in the here and now.

Try this exercise: Take a moment and relax. Focus for a minute on your breathing. Imagine that you are breathing through your heart. If you go to your head and start thinking during the exercise, go back to focusing on your breath and imagine that you are breathing through your heart. Think of something that has made you uncomfortable recently. Let yourself be present with the situation—visualize it again if that helps. Allow whatever feelings there are to arise or be present. Let yourself feel the feelings without judgment or processing. Feel what is happening in your body. Is your body hurting anywhere? What does it feel like in your body, this discomfort? Where is it? Just let yourself feel whatever is there physically or emotionally. Usually some insight will occur, or a sense of relief will occur.

The Underlying Principles of Energy Work

Feeling feelings or doing the above exercise does not make trauma more pronounced, because we are accepting the emotion as we feel it. It is the act of resisting the feelings that creates the trauma. Allowing the feelings with a stance of "it is okay to feel this" allows the body to process the feelings and understand them.

Doing the energy therapies, one will experience emotions much like one does in the above exercise. It is a structured process that allows one to feel emotions and learn from them, gaining insight into our behavior while clearing any trauma that has registered in our system as a fight-or-flight response. The energy therapies help us to be present with and process our emotions. If you are upset and don't know why, often doing an acupressure point or two on the feelings can provide you with more information on the emotions and their origins.

Understanding love and fear

There are only two emotions: love and fear. All of the positive emotions go under the category of love, and all of the negative ones fall into the category of fear. If I feel anger, at the base of that is fear; if I feel joy or peace, the core of that feeling is love. You can choose love or fear. When we are in our "true," aligned state, we are love. Love of self is essential for a positive state of mind. You can only love others as much as you are capable of loving yourself. It is critical to the healing process that we learn to love ourselves and treat ourselves as though we are our own best friends. If we don't, we are most likely reverting back to old patterns that can re-traumatize us to old behaviors.

If we do not love ourselves, we are probably caught in and enforcing negative patterns created by our parents and/or society, and we are limited in our ability to love others. The patterns are the result of their fear, their beliefs, and their negative patterns. For example, a parent may believe that in order to teach you to be a good person, they need to punish you for not conforming to their (or society's) rules. Or they may think they need to be hard on you or you won't learn or be motivated. Or they may just be angry (as a result of their upbringing) and unable or unwilling to control their anger. The constant pattern of our parents' abuse becomes our own pattern when we abuse ourselves with negative self-talk or disapproval.

Often to truly love ourselves, we must clear blocking beliefs that society instills in us.

We are taught that loving the self can lead to a big ego and being selfish. We then deduce that if we are taking care of ourselves, we are selfish, and people won't like us. What a predicament! Energy therapies can remove the traumas and blocking beliefs associated with this negative cycle. Learning to live from our hearts helps us to heal ourselves and it heals others. Literally, living from our heart can heal us and create healing for others. Bringing attention to the heart in times of stress can immediately reduce the stress that our bodies experience (Childre, 1999), thus reducing disease and improving the quality of our lives. Childre has a brilliant methodology for going to the heart when under stress in his book, *The Heartmath Solution*, called "freezeframe."

Another method for practicing self-love is one I have done with many clients. I call it Loving Self Practice:

Sit in a relaxed position, and take a few deep breaths. Imagine that you are breathing from your heart. Imagine that you are held in the chair by some force such as spirit, love, grace, God(dess). Think about someone you love deeply. It could be a child, a pet, or even a material object. Let yourself feel how much you love this person or thing. Imagine that they are in your arms. Now transfer your child-self to your arms and let yourself feel this compassion for your child. Now let yourself feel it for yourself at your current age.

Some find this exercise difficult, so be patient—it may take some practice.

Alignment is critical

If we are aligned, it means we are in line with our values, we live them—we are authentic. We don't just say that we value our family and friends, we deliberately carve out time to spend with them. When we are with them, we are really present, not preoccupied with our next activity. Our behavior demonstrates our values. Alignment means we are connected with ourselves and others, and therefore, we make ethical choices. Acting from an aligned place, we also do what is right for others, because when we are aligned, we are also connected to others with the energy of the field. In this way, we also realize that we actually hurt ourselves when we hurt others. Moreover, when we make poor choices and hurt others we are likely caught in a negative pattern of fear taught to us by our parents or others.

Alignment means that we are in touch with ourselves—we know how we feel, and what supports us, and we face the signals that let us know these things. Alignment means that if we are in a job that is not in line with who we are or who we want to be, that we have the courage to face this truth--and eventually do something about it. In our internal dialogue, we respect ourselves. We do not say we value love and then treat ourselves with anger or hate. If we do this, we do not really value love, and we are not aligned. We are stuck in an old pattern that does not nurture us and saps our creative energy. It is important to acknowledge this pattern and begin to shift it.

If we treat ourselves with impatience and are critical of our own actions, we are not treating ourselves with love. It is healing to practice nurturing ourselves as we would a precious child or our best friend. When you notice you are being critical of yourself, stop. Practice compassion. See the lesson and support yourself in doing it differently next time. Some of us believe that we need to beat ourselves up or we won't remember the lesson. Clear this belief (using CLEAR) and let go of your internal critic.

Alignment is an on-going journey, because as the environment changes, we must also change. Being aligned does not just happen once because we reflected on our values and what we want and how we feel. It is a life-long process of examining where we are now in relation to our feelings, what occurs in our lives, our relationship with others and what we do in the world. Our emotions and our bodies tell us if we are aligned and when we are not. We just need to listen. If we are not aligned, we take action to do something about it.

The power of the past

Our emotions are impacted by our experience with, and our attachments to, our past. These attachments and history can dull our ability to listen to and love ourselves, and thus limits our ability to align ourselves. Understanding the patterns that exist as a result of our past pains and hurts is vital, as these pains inhibit our ability to live in the here and now. Moreover, they stimulate stress just by just thinking about traumatic events because the fight-or-flight-immobility response is ignited. For example, I may have a defensive reaction to someone in a position of authority telling me what to do. When someone says, "Don't do that," and I automatically want to fight back and rebel I am not in the present. It is my past that guides my reaction and I may not even know what the present situation demands.

However, if I am truly present to the person speaking in the situation I will know if I need to reject the advice or embrace it as helpful wisdom. To make this decision, I must actually hear it. If I am reacting from a place of rebellion then I cannot be present in the moment to listen and then respond in a new way. I am reacting from my history and patterns. Reacting from history and patterns reduces our options and creativity. Typically, this response is predictable and ineffective in creating real relationships.

Our pains and patterns can be understood and released using the energy therapies. When we release them, we can see and feel more clearly and are therefore more present. And we are free to love ourselves, live in our hearts, and have a spiritual connection.

Becoming conscious of our impact

It is impossible not to have an impact in the world. Knowing this, and knowing that we are all connected, it is important to be aware of what we do and how our actions impact others and the universe. Awareness creates responsibility and choice. It requires observation of and honesty to ourselves and to others regarding what we see and feel. Since objective observation of what we see is not possible, the more we understand our past and how it impacts us and our feelings, the more we understand how we project that past onto the present—and consequently distort it. In altering the present in this way, we create more chaos and less cohesion for ourselves and for those around us. If we clear our past using the energy therapies, we see reality more clearly, and have less negative impact on those around us.

Our interactions with others impact us, and they impact others. Who we associate with affects us. Take an obvious example: when someone quits drugs, alcohol or an old way of being, they usually need to change the groups with which they interact or their changes won't last. The old system has not changed; thus going back into the dysfunctional group draws the person back into old behavior. Another example is a classic phenomena called parallel process, which exists when other parts of a group mirror the tension or conflict at the highest levels of the system. Research has shown, for example, that patients in a psychiatric ward are more violent when there is conflict occurring among the staff. So it greatly benefits us to be aware not only of our impact, but also the impact of others upon us. If that impact is not what we desire, then we need to change. Change comes about through becoming aware of how the past impacts us and clearing traumas that block our desired behavior.

Illuminating the energetic body

Everything has an energetic body that is impacted by its physical, spiritual, and (if appropriate) emotional states. Understanding the condition of our energetic body facilitates an understanding of how to align with our spirit and our soul purpose. Our energy reflects our state of mind, spirit, and physical body, and our state of mind, spirit, and physical body impact what occurs with our energy.

Systems, groups, and organizations also have an energetic body which can also be understood and aligned. The energy of those around us influences us. Awareness is critical if we want to maintain ourselves and our alignment when we are in the presence of others who are not aligned. Working with our energy and seeing that it stays aligned in these situations helps to reduce negative influence.

Imagine that your energy is a luminous egg that fills your body and then continues out beyond the body about a foot and a half. This energy egg is impacted by our daily experiences. Interactions can cause us to retract our energy or pull it behind us so that it is no longer centered around the body. This causes stress on the system. I have felt energy to the side of people, below them, to the right of them, reaching out to one side. The variations are endless. The point is that all of the variations other than the centered one are stressful and prevent us from being fully present.

Being able to sense your energy (whether you see it or feel it) may take some practice, but is not necessary to create a feeling of being centered and grounded. Bringing the energy back to center is simple. Do the waterfall exercise in Appendix D, or just see if you can sense your field. Feel where it is, and create the intention to bring it back to center, imagining it filling out like a balloon from your heart and ending about a foot or so beyond your body. You can also smooth the energy by gently rubbing it in an upward movement like you are polishing an egg.

Sometimes the energy body refuses to move back to this position because of past trauma; the person feels it is not safe to be fully present. The energy therapies help the body feel safe enough to bring the field back, especially if there is severe trauma and disassociation.

The fundamental paradoxes by which we evolve

The dichotomy of life creates our understanding of life. Our sadness, anger or discomfort help us to understand and know happiness, love and comfort. These paradoxes provide us with the understanding we need to evolve, just as Jesus and Saddam Hussein give us dichotomous options for being human. Understanding the dichotomy provides us with choice, provided we are "conscious." If we are not conscious, then we just react to situations we don't like, because we are unable to see the lessons in the dichotomy. Looking at what we can learn from a situation is critical in reframing it from one that is sometimes unbearable to one that has merit.

I have one client who offers a great example of finding a wonderful lesson in dichotomy. This woman was devastated when her husband left her. Initially, she struggled with her will to live, but a year later she has found her passion in her work, and gone down a path that is incredibly rewarding—one she would not have found had she remained married. She feels more in touch with herself and her purpose than she ever did before her divorce. She now frames the split as a blessing, although at the time it was the most difficult experience she had ever been through.

Life is full of difficulty and hate—and also, hopefully, love and joy. All of these things make up life. Often we strive to better ourselves so that we just have the joy, the peace and contentment. This is not the goal of healing. The goal of healing is to accept and be present with the joy and the pain, to be in relationship with ourselves and with others.

We are all evolving

We are all attempting to evolve. It is natural to grow and change. It is also natural to want comfort. Where we can get stuck is in the attempt to stay comfortable by ignoring the signals indicating that change could benefit us. Encourage continual learning for yourself and for others. Challenge the need to be comfortable and find ways to support your growth and learning. It is possible to be content in all of it. In order to do this, we have to get "out" of ourselves; we need to observe ourselves, practice not taking ourselves so seriously, and see our connection to others and spirit, meditate, and understand death, for then we can appreciate all of life. Observe the learnings and the positives experienced through the difficult. Be thankful for the difficulties and resulting lessons—and heal our stuck traumas.

APPENDIX C
Specific Blocking Beliefs

As I have worked with clients over the years, I created and added to these lists of blocking beliefs. If an issue is not clearing, review the list related to the issue and muscle test them to see if there are either beliefs or traumas you need to clear. Though they are called blocking beliefs, and we usually use the sore points to clear such beliefs there are often other points to clear besides the sore points. You may also use the list to check for specific issues to clear.

Being in love blocking beliefs
Love will save me.
If he/she doesn't want me, then I'm not loveable.
If I want him/her then he/she should want me.
I can't believe that he/she doesn't love me.
I have to have someone in love with me to be acceptable.
I have to be in love to be happy.
Being in love is the only thing worth doing.
Being in love is the main reason to be here.
Being in love is the only thing that can make me happy.
Being in love is the main reason to be alive.
Being in love makes me whole.
Being in love is what makes me a human.
Being in love is the most important thing in life.
Being in love gives me a reason to be alive.
Love is the only thing worth living for.

Love is the only thing that matters.
There will never be anyone else like him/her.
There is only one true love.
We only get one chance.
If she/he doesn't want me then there is something wrong with me.
If I heal this trauma, then it will destroy my view of true love.
If I don't have love then I am nothing.
Love is forever.
We should be true forever.
I'll lose anyone I love.

Belonging blocking beliefs
I don't belong.
Everyone hates me.
Life is hard/life is wonderful.
No one sees me (I am invisible).
No one values me.
I am lost.
I am uncomfortable.
People don't care about me.
I am alone.
I am unwanted.
I am forgotten.
I am insecure.
I am unlovable.

Connection blocking beliefs
It is not safe to connect with others.
I can't determine with whom it is safe to connect.
I will be hurt if I connect with others.
It is not possible to connect with others.

Specific Blocking Beliefs

I don't want to connect with others.
I will be hurt if I connect with others.
It is dangerous to connect with others.
Others will find out how deficient I am if I connect.
Others will see all of my faults if we connect.
Others will not want to be with me if we connect.
I will have to be responsible to this person if I connect with him/her.

Female blocking beliefs

I should give him what he wants.
I have an obligation to give him sex.
I have to take care of everyone.
A woman's job is to take care of everyone.
A woman is "less than" a man.
A woman should do what the man wants.
Women should downplay their strength.
Women are weaker.
My anger is bad.
Anger is not okay for women.
Happiness is the only acceptable emotion.
I'm a bitch if I'm angry.
Women are emotional and irrational.
Men are the brains.
Men are more capable.
Men are stronger.
My emotions make me weaker.
My emotions make me "less than."
Men should control women.
Men are stronger.
Men are better.
I should be pure for him.

I have to be "lady-like."
I shouldn't be powerful.

Male blocking beliefs [females may have these also]
It's not okay to feel my fear.
It's not okay to have emotions.
I'll be a wimp if I cry.
It's not okay to cry.
I'll be a wimp if I have emotions.
It's not okay to feel.
I can't feel.
I can't be a good man and feel my feelings.
I'll lose control if I feel my feelings.
It's not safe to feel my feelings.
I don't want to feel my feelings.
I have to be strong.
I can't be vulnerable and be strong.
I won't be seen as strong if I am vulnerable or if I cry.
I should be the one in control.

Money blocking beliefs
Money is the root of all evil.
You can't have money and be spiritual.
If you have money, you are greedy.
If you want to be rich, you are selfish.
I don't know how to handle money.
If you have money then you aren't a good person.
Money is dirty.
If you have more than enough money, then you aren't a good person.
I deserve lots of money.
It's possible to have lots of money.

Specific Blocking Beliefs

I am smart enough to have lots of money.
I have what it takes to make lots of money.
You have to work really hard to make lots of money.
It is difficult to make lots of money.
People won't like me if I have lots of money.
I won't be able to tell who are my real friends if I have lots of money.
Making lots of money is too much effort/too much work.
I will be judged/criticized/shamed if I have lots of money.
I don't deserve to enjoy/possess the good/beautiful things in life.

Over-responsibility

I have to work to justify my existence/I can let the beauty I love be what I do.
I have to work to justify my existence/My existence needs no justification.
I do lots of things I don't enjoy because I feel I should/I don't have to do what I don't enjoy just because I feel I should.
I must take care of my obligations and responsibilities before anything else/I can make room for beauty, play, and pleasure in my life.
I am responsible for everyone and everything/I am responsible only for myself.
I am responsible for everyone's actions/I am responsible only for my actions.
I am responsible for other adults' actions/I am not responsible for other adults' actions.
I take responsibility for others' growth/I take responsibility only for my own growth.
I take responsibility for others' consciousness/I take responsibility only for my own consciousness.
I take responsibility for the care of others' bodies/I take responsibility only for the care of my body.
I take responsibility for the care of others' psyche/I take responsibility only for the care of my psyche.
I take responsibility for the care of others' spirit/I take responsibility only for the care of my spirit.
I take full responsibility for how my relationships go/I take responsibility for how I treat people.

Religion-related blocking beliefs

I was born in original sin.
I need to be punished/I deserve to be punished.
I don't deserve to be loved.
I am evil.
I have done evil things.
I did bad things.
I am a bad person.
I am a hateful person.
I can never be forgiven.
I can't forgive myself.
God doesn't love me.
God will never forgive me.
I am not worthy of God's love.
I am a sinner.
I can never be saved.
I have sinned and can't be forgiven.
I can't be a good person no matter how hard I try.
It's virtuous to be in pain.
I have to suffer to be a good person/get God's blessing.
I have to do penance.
I have to suffer to do penance.
It's blasphemous to be psychic.
The occult is evil.
Practicing the occult means you are in cahoots with the devil.

Relationship blocking beliefs

It is safe to be in relationship.
I trust others.
I shouldn't trust people.
People are not trustworthy.

Specific Blocking Beliefs

People aren't safe.
I'm not safe with others.
If I love, I will get hurt.
I don't want to be close to people.
I want love/I don't want love.
I deserve love/to be loved.

Responsibility blocking beliefs

I do lots of things I don't enjoy because I feel I should.
I am responsible for everyone and everything.
I am responsible for others' feelings.
I am responsible for everyone's actions.
I am responsible for the problems of others.

Self-love blocking beliefs

I should/shouldn't take care of myself.
It is safe to take care of myself.
I should think of others and not myself.
I am selfish if I think of myself.
I love myself/I hate myself.
I should/shouldn't love myself.
If I love myself, I will have a big head.
I want to love myself.
It is egotistical to love myself.
Others won't like me if I love myself.
I won't be thinking of others if I do it for myself.

Work and success blocking beliefs

I am incapable.
I am stupid/I am smart.
I have to work to justify my existence.

I have to work hard to be successful.
It's not possible for me to be successful.
I have to do a lot to be accepted.
I don't have what it takes to be successful.
I don't deserve to be successful.
I will misuse my power if I am successful.
It is safe to use my power.
I am powerful.

APPENDIX D
Useful Exercises

The waterfall exercise
Try recording this on a CD or on an audio tape, so that you can follow along to your own voice.

> Close your eyes. Feel yourself relax. Breath in and out deeply a few times. Ask yourself where there are blocks in your body—identify those places. Let a waterfall begin to flow down through your head, down through your body and down through your feet. It is a warm bubbly waterfall. And as it flows through, it goes to the dark areas of blockages and the bubbles carry the darkness away out through the body and down through the feet and into the ground. Let this continue for a few minutes until you feel clear of blocks, relaxed and calm. Then imagine a clear, white, healing light coming up from your feet, up through your legs, up through the torso and out through the top of your head. Then bring your energy fully into your heart, let it expand out into your whole body and then into the energy sphere beyond your body, about a foot and a half. When you feel ready, come back to the room and open your eyes.

Being present in your body
This exercise helps you to be present in the here and now and is good to do before working with a client or doing acupressure point work on yourself.

> Sit in a comfortable position with both of your feet on the ground, and close your eyes. Take a few deep breaths and feel your body. Let yourself sink down into the seat and feel your butt on the chair. Imagine that you are breathing through your

heart. Let your focus stay there for a while. Then let yourself be aware of all of the different parts of your body. Focus on legs. See if there is any tension there. Just let yourself be aware of how it feels, without consciously trying to change it, but observe any changes that occur. Then move up to your stomach area. What does it feel like? Is there any tension? Is there any information in the tension? Then move up to the chest and check in there. Repeat with the shoulders, arms, neck, and head. Slowly come back to the room and open your eyes.

Breathing through the heart

Try this exercise: Take a moment and relax. Focus for a minute on your breathing. Imagine that you are breathing through your heart. If you go to your head and start thinking during the exercise, go back to focusing on your breath and imagine that you are breathing through your heart. Think of something that has made you uncomfortable recently. Let yourself be present with the situation—visualize it again if that helps. Allow whatever feelings there are to arise or be present. Let yourself feel the feelings without judgment or processing. Feel what is happening in your body. Is your body hurting anywhere? What does it feel like in your body, this discomfort? Where is it? Just let yourself feel whatever is there physically or emotionally. Usually some insight will occur, or a sense of relief will occur.

Loving self practice

Another method for practicing self-love is one I have done with many clients. I call it Loving Self Practice:

Sit in a relaxed position, and take a few deep breaths. Imagine that you are breathing from your heart. Imagine that you are held in the chair by some force such as spirit, love, grace, God(dess). Think about someone you love deeply. It could be a child, a pet, or even a material object. Let yourself feel how much you love this person or thing. Imagine that they are in your arms. Now transfer your child-self to your arms and let yourself feel this compassion for your child. Now let yourself feel it for yourself at your current age.

Some find this exercise difficult, so be patient—it may take some practice.

APPENDIX E
Issues Cleared

I generated the following issues from my work with friends, colleagues and students who do the energy therapies on themselves. I hope it provides additional ideas about the kinds of issues you can work on, besides those I have covered elsewhere in the book.

Work and career
    I am afraid of being powerful or successful; I can't handle the responsibility.
    If I dedicate myself to work, I'll drown.
    If I am successful, I have to be strong and I can't be vulnerable or soft.
    The reward for hard work is more hard work.
    I can't have impact in the world and be myself, be a woman.
    I'm too young to be successful.
    I'm not supposed to do what I want to do (it's not worthwhile).
    If I'm competent, then I'm cold.
    If I'm warm and soft, then I'm not competent.
    I have to be stressed to be successful.
    Being successful is hard work.

Self-concept
    I have to be perfect.
    I have to do something to be valuable.
    I can't have it all or do it all.
    I don't have enough energy.
    I need to impress people or they won't like me.

I'm not enough.
People don't want me to be who I am.
If I say "no," people won't like me or I'll cause conflict.
Being educated takes away my ability to be myself.

Family issues

My mother is sick, so there will be something wrong with me; it's in my genes.
I'm afraid I will be like my mother/father.
I need to feel other's emotions so that I know what they are thinking and can stay safe.
If I forgive him, I let him off the hook and I'll get hurt again.
I need to/want to get sick when there is conflict so I can avoid it.
My mother wants me to be different.
My parents are angry so there must be something wrong with me; if I could be different, they wouldn't be angry with me.
They all hate me.
They don't want me.
I want them to take care of me (neglect).

Relationships

I don't have time for relationships.
If I love someone, I'll lose him/her.
I'll be betrayed.
I don't want a relationship—I'll just be hurt again.

Emotions

I don't want conflict, negative feelings, and discomfort.
I don't want my feelings (guilt, anger, pain, sadness).
I need drama or I'm not alive.
If I am really emotional, people will pay attention to me.

Issues Cleared

Sex
    I'm not sexy.
    I don't want to be sexy.
    If I'm not skinny, I'm not sexy.
    I have shame around sex (it's dirty).

Sleep
    I can't sleep.
    It's too dangerous to sleep.
    It's a waste of time to sleep.
    If I sleep, I'll have nightmares.
    If I sleep, someone will hurt me.

Miscellaneous
    Society expects me to have children.
    I don't want to leave home; I get stressed from traveling.
    There is never enough time.
    There's never enough.
    If I complete something, I'll be judged.
    I'm afraid of death (from the trauma of death of a family member, friend, relative or pet).

Bibliography

Andrade, Joaquin, M.D. and Feinstein, David, Ph.D.
"Preliminary Report of the First Large-Scale Study of Energy Psychology."
http://www.nolimiteftbooks.com/members/1551023/uploaded/EPStudy.pdf, 2003.

Childre, Doc and Martin, Howard.
The Heartmath Solution.
San Francisco: Harper, 1999.

Chopra, Deepak, M.D.
Ageless Body, Timeless Mind.
New York: Harmony Books, 1993.

Feinstein, David; Eden, Donna; and Craig, Gary.
The Promise of Energy Psychology.
New York: Jeremy P. Tarcher/Penguin, 2005.

Jensen, Derrick.
A Language Older than Words.
Vermont: Chelsea Green Publishing, 2004.

Johnson, Steven.
Mind Wide Open: Your Brain and the Neuroscience of Everyday Life.
New York: Scribner, 2004.

Levine, Peter.
"Healing Trauma, Restoring the Wisdom of Your Body."
Audio tape. Boulder: Sounds True, 1999.

Levoy, Gregg.
Callings: Finding and Following an Authentic Life.
New York: Three Rivers Press, 1997.

McTaggart, Lynne.
The Field, the Quest for the Secret Force of the Universe.
New York: HarperCollins Publishers, 2002.

Ruden, Ronald A., M.D., Ph.D.
Why Tapping Works: Speculations from the Observable Brain.
http://energypsych.org/article-ruden2.php, 2005.

Talbot, Michael. *The Holographic Universe.*
New York: HarperCollins, 1991.

About the Author

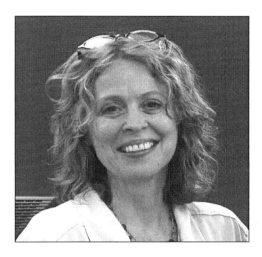

Julie Roberts, Ph.D.

Julie Roberts consults with organizations and individuals to help them move into their full potential. She specializes in personal, professional, and organizational change, so individuals and groups overcome obstacles to productivity. Using energy therapies, muscle testing, visualization and counseling, she assists people in clearing the blocks in their life. She also teaches graduate courses and workshops to train others in her energy psychology, improve their leadership skills, and guide individuals through a healing change process. Julie lives in rural Pennsylvania near Philadelphia. www.changeworksinc.com